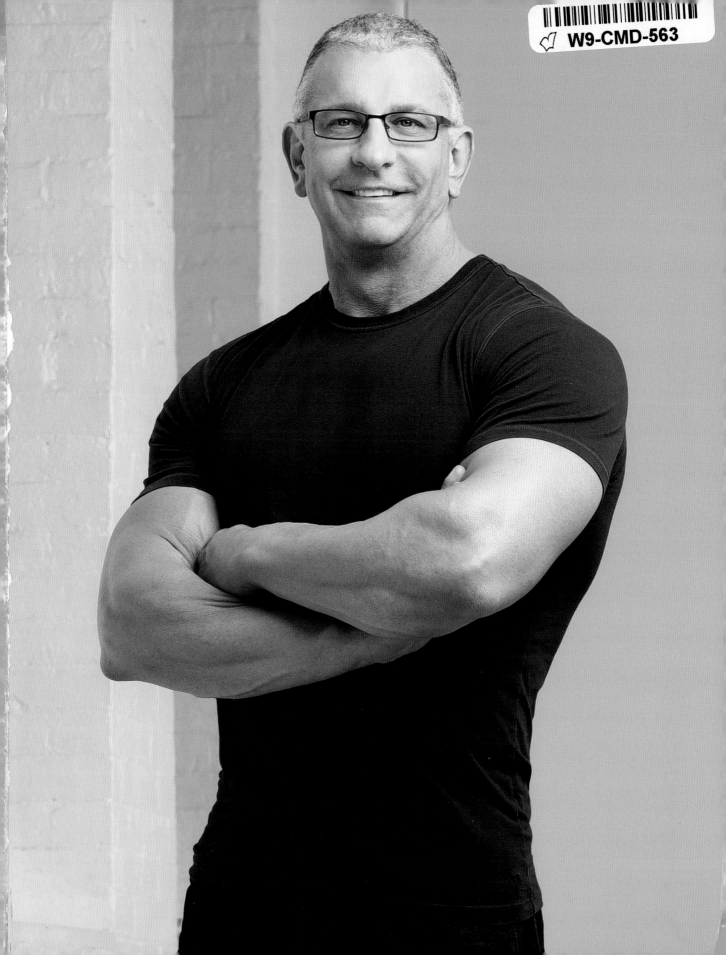

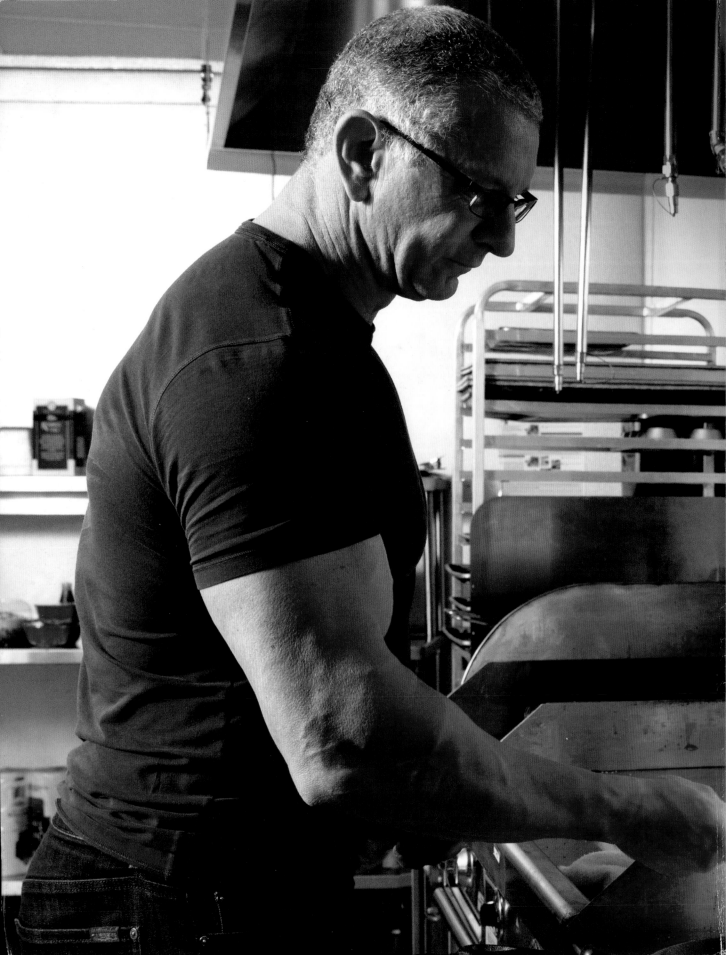

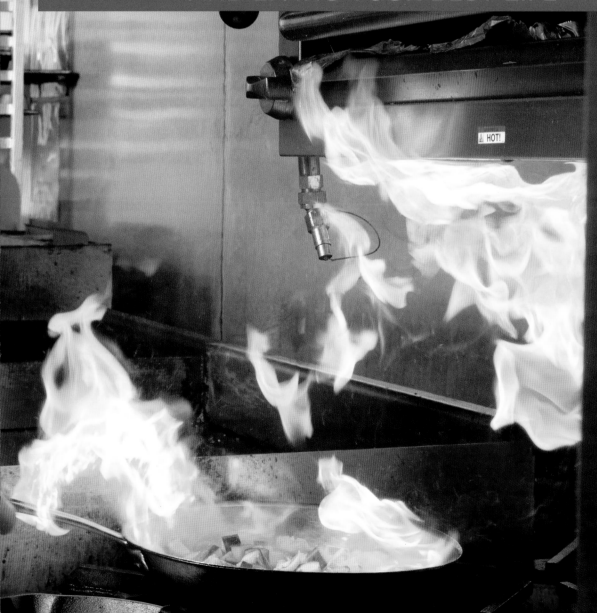

FIT FUEL

A CHEF'S GUIDE TO EATING WELL, GETTING FIT, AND LIVING YOUR BEST LIFE

HOT!

Third printing, 2016

ISBN: 978-0-9964223-0-7 (Hardcover)
ISBN: 978-0-9964223-1-4 (Paperback)

Irvine Products, LLC
1227 N. Franklin St.
Tampa, FL 33602

chefirvine.com

Creative Direction and Design: Sean Otto

Photography: Ian Spanier

Food shot on location at:
Rat's Restaurant at Grounds for Sculpture, Yardley, PA

Page 47 image courtesy of Lee South
Page 23 image courtesy of Dave Burrows/Shutterstock.com
Page 103 image courtesy of Julie Clopper/Shutterstock.com
Pages 12, 14, 19, 21, 28, 32, 36, 38, 40, 45, 46, 50, 97, 98, 101, 105
 courtesy of Shutterstock.com

For Gail,

who makes me want to get the most out of life every day.

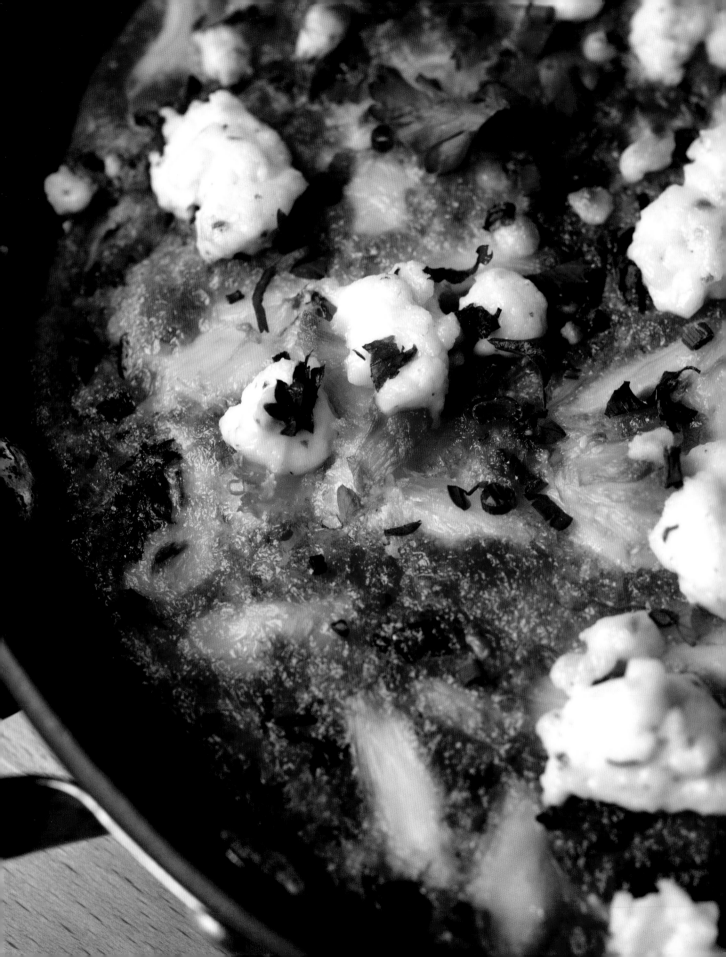

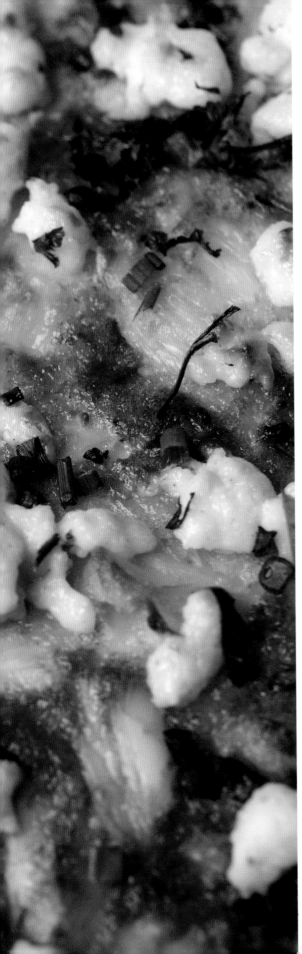

CONTENTS

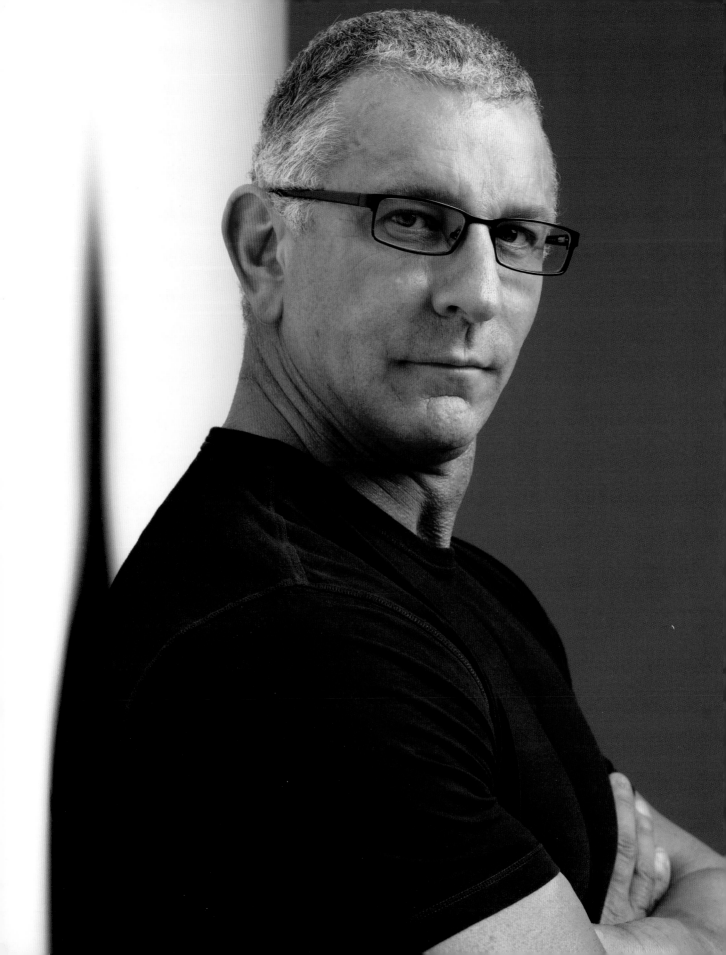

Why I Wrote This Book

The overabundance of fitness information available today has made you skeptical of new books—and of their authors. I don't blame you.

TO START, YOU HAVE QUESTIONS THAT NEED ANSWERING. For example:

Why would you write this book now?

There are a lot of healthy chefs promoting their recipes. Why should I listen to you?

So many superfit models and self-styled gurus offer their own branded training programs—how is yours any different?

This is my answer:

I've made every health and fitness mistake a man can make. I've eaten like crap, fallen into a lazy routine with the gym, and paid the price with my own health. I'll tell that story in the coming pages. For now, what you need to know is that I'm not someone who was "born with it." I didn't grow up instinctively knowing how to train. I didn't have a natural talent for cooking that ran in my family. (In fact, as you'll learn, it was quite the opposite.) And even once I'd learned how to cook, I didn't know a damn thing about how to make meals that would keep me healthy or fit.

And yet, I've been able to put it all together in a way few others ever have. Look at every fitness model in the world, and I guarantee you that not one of them can cook like I can. Take all the greatest chefs in the world, and I guarantee you not one of them looks like me, or is capable of doing what I can in the gym. Today I am truly blessed with the best of both worlds: I'm healthy and fit, but I make absolutely no compromises when it comes to food.

Plain broccoli and chicken? The fitness models and bodybuilders can keep it. I'm never going to eat that way, and you don't have to, either.

I am a classic example of someone who had to learn every single lesson the hard way—and now I've written this book so you don't have to.

You don't have to repeat the mistakes I've made. You don't have to beat your head against the wall, thinking you're doing the right things but worrying something's wrong with you because you can't lose fat and build muscle.

If you had told me just a few short years ago that, at 50 years old, I'd appear on the cover of a fitness magazine, shirtless and with a visible six-pack, I would have said you were absolutely insane. Yet I did just that. Such is the power of the lessons I learned through failure. The book you now hold in your hands is the result of those lessons, and you can use it to turn your life around.

Learn to train smart and safe—but with intensity. Learn to cook healthy but delicious food. Learn to redefine what's possible for you. Banish doubt once and for all. You *can* have it all. Because if I can do it, anyone can do it. It's truly not that difficult. The finer points of training and cooking—anyone can learn those. Let me be your teacher.

But first, you must begin by believing that it's possible for you to change in a major way. There is a power inside you that you don't even know you have. Let's discover it together.

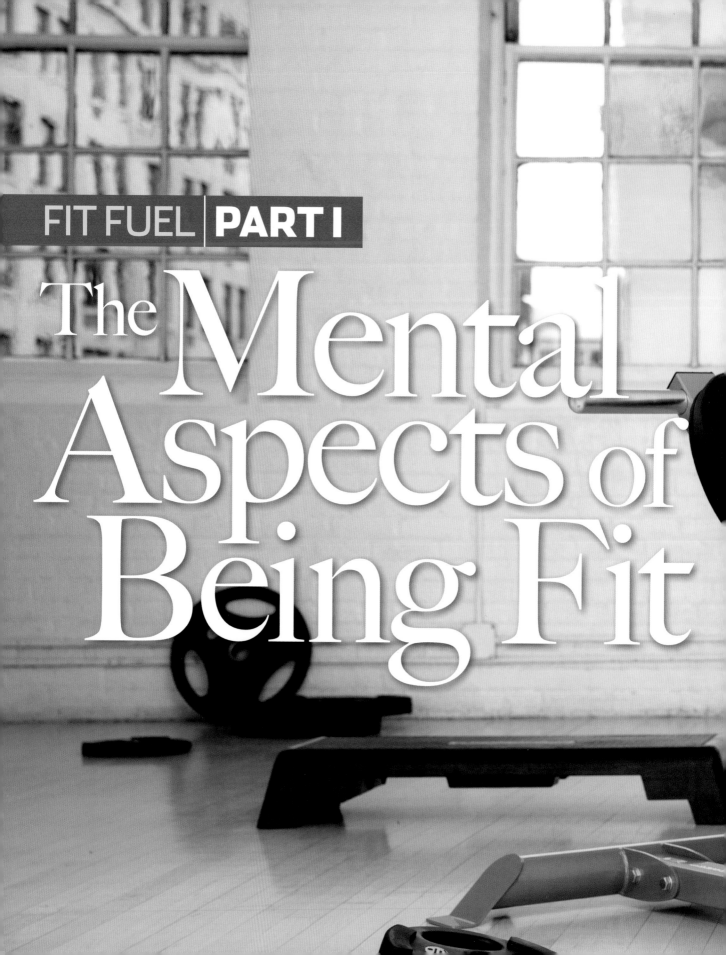

FIT FUEL | **PART I**

The Mental Aspects of Being Fit

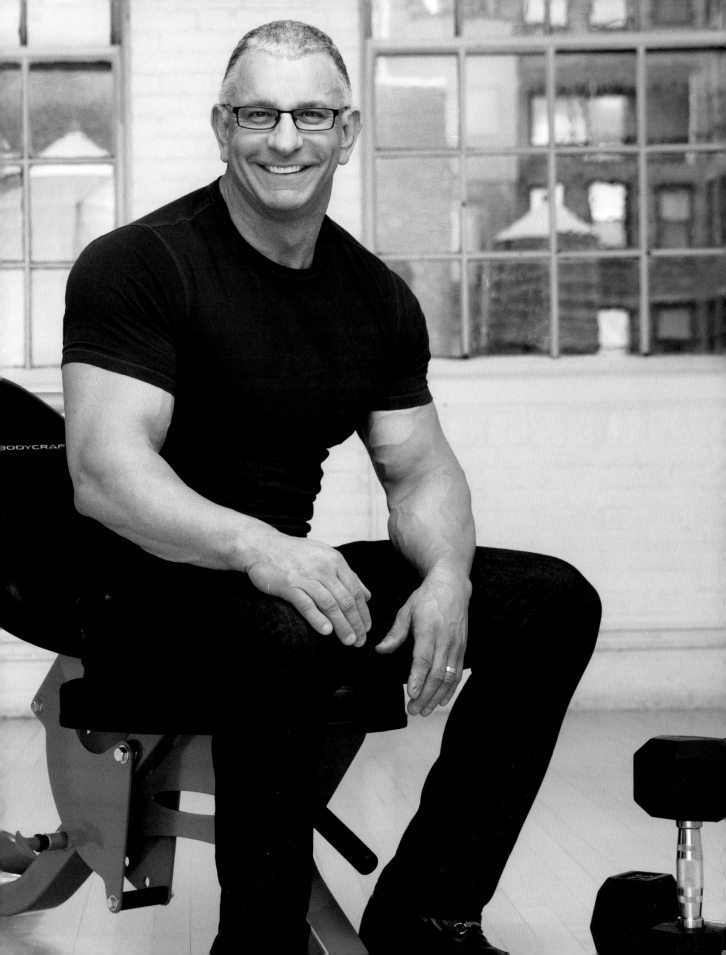

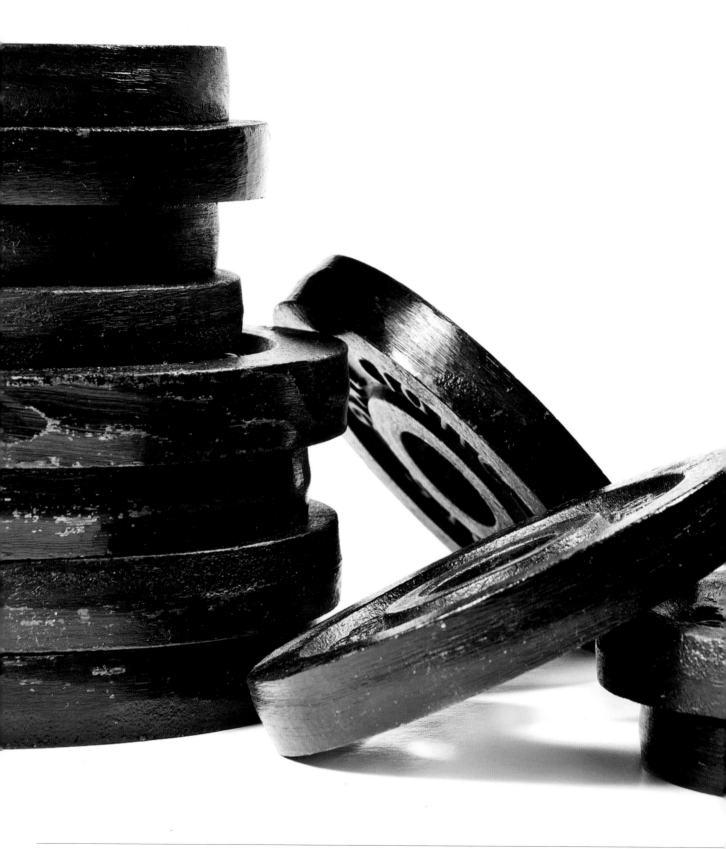

What Fitness Means to Me

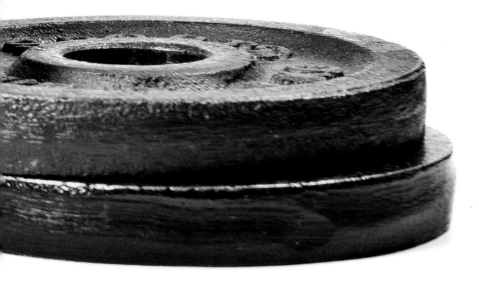

I LOVE THE FITNESS LIFESTYLE. I love working out—the way it makes me feel, and the knowledge that what I'm doing is keeping me healthy. I truly believe that a membership at a good gym and a solid training program comprise the best healthcare plan you can ever have. Over the years I have fully integrated training and healthy eating into my lifestyle. Since I travel about 300 days a year, this isn't always easy, but I make it work because it's a priority. Here's what living a fit lifestyle means to me.

IT MEANS BEING DEDICATED, BUT NOT OBSESSED

My morning gym session with the crew of one of my shows is as much a part of my daily routine as taking a shower or eating breakfast. It's part of who I am. But as much as I love to work out, I would not categorize myself as obsessed. And when I say that, I make no judgments on those who *are* fitness-obsessed. For people who live to work out, that's their prerogative; and as far as obsessions go, it's a wonderful thing to live for something that can only improve your health.

But to me, being fit isn't an end in itself—it's something that empowers the other passions in life, whatever they may be. Being fit means I can keep up with a travel and filming schedule that would decimate a man in lesser shape, yet still have energy left over to put into maintaining quality relationships with my wife and family. You may not travel as much as I do, but I'm sure you have comparable stressors in your life—family, job responsibilities, things to fix around the house, etc.—that could open the door to all sorts of unhealthy eating habits and the chronic illnesses that could follow. Being fit will help you meet those life challenges.

I make this distinction to show you that your life doesn't have to be a hardline choice between being sedentary and being all-out fitness-obsessed. You can be fit and healthy without spending all day worrying about when you're going to get back to the gym for a second cardio session.

You can do it all without letting it take over your life. That's what this book is all about.

IT MEANS HAVING A PLAN—AND A WILLINGNESS TO FOLLOW THROUGH

My work schedule is never planned more than a few weeks in advance. Once I do know where I'm going, however, the first priority is to find a gym for our crew training sessions. It's not always easy to wake up in some strange hotel room and get out the door to start exercising in a brand-new gym, but we do it together and it brings us all closer. It gives us the feeling of being with family, and a sense of normalcy.

Moreover, the impact on our overall health is phenomenal. Too many people who have to travel a lot for business simply throw in the towel at the very idea of fitness, thinking it's far too much of a bother to keep up with. If I didn't have a reliable plan of attack every time I hit the gym, I might think it was pointless, too. But I don't wander in and try to think of something new each day. I have a specific training template I work from—the very template that has helped me build the big arms I'm known for (about 21 inches, to be precise, thank you very much) while keeping my body fat low enough that I have visible abs year-round.

It might seem vain for me to talk about myself in such terms, I know, but the fact of the matter is this: If you look in the mirror and are proud of what you see, that carries over into every other facet of daily life. If you look good, you feel good; and if you feel good all the time, there's no limit to what you can accomplish in life. In this book I'm going to provide you with my training template, organized into an easy-to-follow chart that will make it simple for you to effect radical changes in your body.

If you're looking for one-off workouts that can be done when you're short on time, I've got you covered there, too. More than anyone else, I think I understand the value of having a Plan B for those days when your schedule just isn't conducive to a full hour-plus session in the gym. In this one-off section, I'm going to share with you the best time-saving workouts I've ever come up with.

So far I've used words like "simple" and "easy-to-follow," and of course all that is true. But I'm not going to lie to you: This is going to require a lot of hard work on your part. Just as there's no magic pill that can give you a six-pack, there's no book that can make you fit, either. The secret ingredient that's going to make this work is your own sweat. Trust in the program and apply intensity to the techniques I'm giving you and success *will* follow.

IT MEANS PREPARING HEALTHY FOODS WITHOUT SACRIFICING FLAVOR

You should know that it wasn't always easy for me to cook healthy meals.

If you're a chef, the food you make isn't judged on whether or not it's healthy. In my profession, flavor always has and always will trump any other factor. Creativity, plating, and the dining atmosphere you create for your patrons are all considered more important than the nutritional value of your dishes. So it's tempting to fall back on sugar, fat, and salt, because they

all have a powerful impact on the taste buds—and, in the hands of the right chef, can help turn a good dish into a truly memorable one. (If you know of an easier way to quickly thicken up a sauce than with a hefty dollop of butter or a few tablespoons of cornstarch, I'd love to hear it!)

But the more I wrestled with this concept (and my own health issues, as you'll learn later), the more it became a real dilemma for me—especially as I began to realize that the obesity epidemic had spiraled into a world health catastrophe. I resolved not to add extra fat, sugar, or salt to a recipe if there was a better way of developing the flavors I wanted to come out of that particular dish. I didn't swear off these elements entirely, nor do I think you should. I distrust any diet or nutritional philosophy that says you can *never* eat certain things, just as I distrust any fad diet that deletes an entire macronutrient—think of the recent no-carb craze, or, in the '80s, the no-fat craze. Insanity!

Crossing a bunch of foods off the list of what you can eat is a practice destined to fail. If you've ever done this, then you need to learn to stop thinking of food in those terms and start thinking of it in terms of habits that will make you successful. Your approach has to be less about saying no to greasy fast food and more about saying yes to learning to enjoy vegetables, fruit, and lean protein. With this book I'm giving you the road map for getting there.

If you follow my cooking tips and recipes, you will see the best possible change you could ever ask for: You will begin to truly crave healthy and nutritious food. This change will take hold soon after you learn that you can eat flavorful, satisfying dishes at every meal and walk away from the table without feeling like you might roll down the street. The regret that sets in after a heavy meal is almost immediate. We're going to do away with that feeling for good, and replace it with great food that will give you the energy you need to attack life and get everything you want out of it.

Of course, this isn't to say you can never have an actual cheat meal. As much as anyone, I love a good dessert. There absolutely is a time and a place for some cheating—but to earn it, you've got to do some serious training (yes, back to training!). You have to work out and deplete your muscles to the point where they're ready to soak up some of the extra calories you consume afterward. In the meal-planning section of this book, some of the desserts and the more calorically dense meals are intended specifically to fall on such intense-training days, and are labeled as such.

And in the end, isn't that better than some magic pill? Search deep in your memory and think of all the times you got something for

nothing. How did you feel about it? Did you value it as much as something you had worked day and night for? When you think about things you earned through hard work versus those you got at practically no cost, it's not hard to figure out why so many people who get liposuction, Lap-Band surgery, or gastric bypass surgery often fall right back into the unhealthy habits that got them into such dire straits in the first place.

IT MEANS FALLING BACK IN LOVE WITH FOOD—AND NEVER FEELING GUILTY AGAIN

If you're like me, or any of the millions of people who watch the Food Network every day, you look at food as not just nutrition but as a way of connecting with your past and present, a way to bring your family together, to be social, to celebrate. Food nourishes not just the body, but the heart, mind, and soul. However, this doesn't change the fact that, to your body, food is fuel for its engine—nothing more and nothing less. How well that engine runs is directly determined by what type of fuel you put into it.

I've developed recipes for foods your body can use as high-octane fuel *and* that you can enjoy on all the secondary levels—recipes that taste so good they'll remind you of why you fell in love with food in the first place. Now I want you to fall in love with it all over again—but never feel guilty about it.

A chef's dishes are judged on flavor, not on nutritional value. But I resolved to find better ways to develop flavor than simply adding extra fat, sugar, or salt.

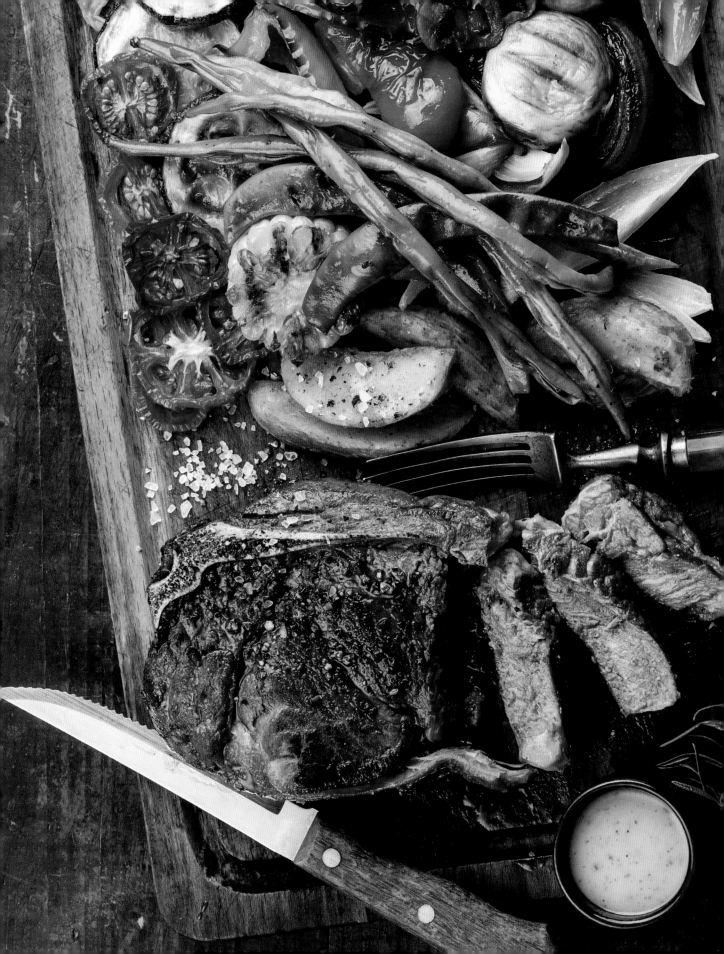

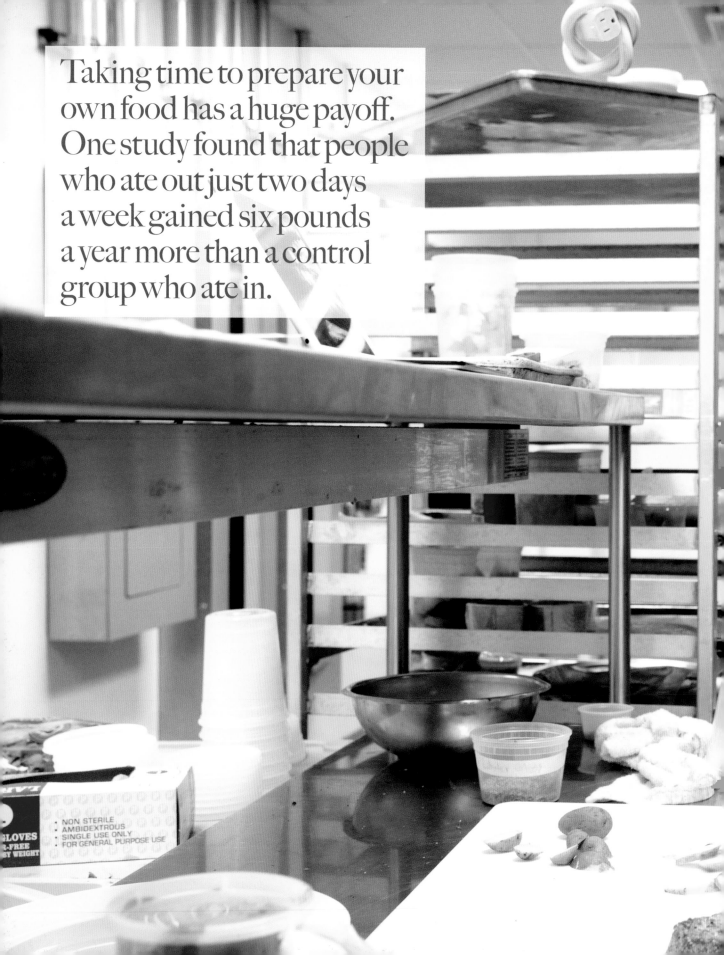

Taking time to prepare your own food has a huge payoff. One study found that people who ate out just two days a week gained six pounds a year more than a control group who ate in.

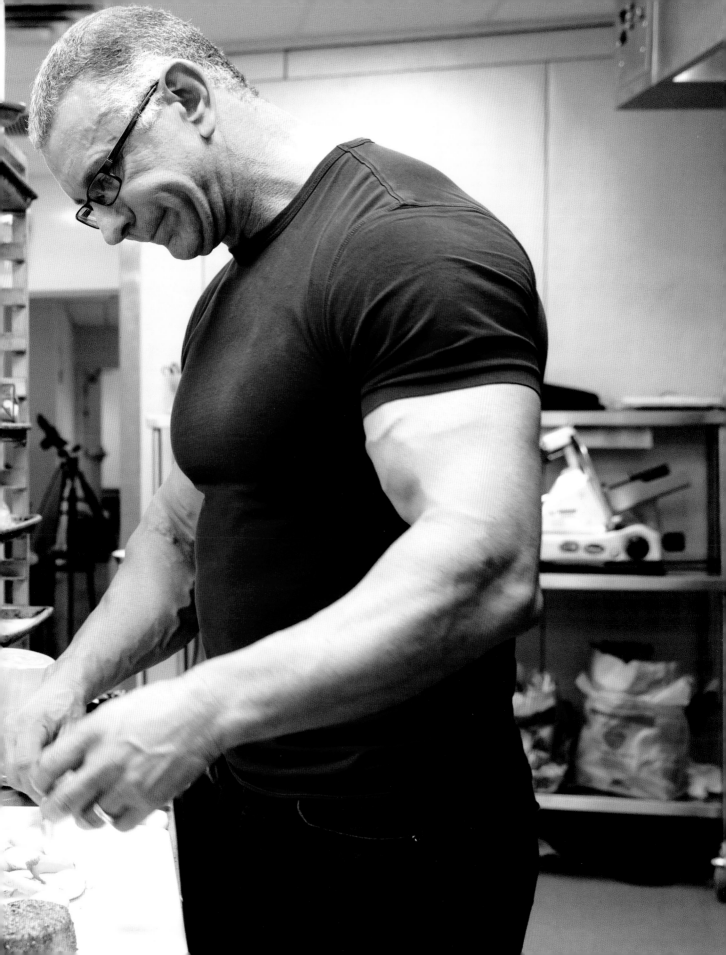

Life, or How I Got to Where I Am Today

In a nutshell, it goes something like this...

I GREW UP IN A THREE-BEDROOM council flat in Crumpsall, Manchester, England. It was me, my mother, Patricia, my father, Walter, my brother, Gary, and my sisters Colleen and Jackie. It was a modest home for people of modest means, but within those walls we had love and support—everything we needed to make our dreams come true.

A SCRAWNY KID WITH A CRAZY DREAM

My dream was to become a bodybuilder... Okay, so it didn't exactly come true. But pursuing it set me on a path to having everything I ever wanted—all of my career success can be traced back to chasing that dream.

I'll dive into that in a second. First, I think it's time I let you know something you don't know about me, something I've never spoken about in public: My mother and father divorced when I was about 6 years old. I probably never told anyone before because if you had ever run into my parents, you'd never have known they were divorced.

The "split," after all, happened more than 40 years ago, yet Walter and Pat lived together until he died in the fall of 2014. At the time of the divorce, my dad did move out—but he came back about 10 weeks later. They reconciled, and every Sunday after that he asked my mum to marry him again. She said no every time, but he kept asking. If you've ever watched an episode of *Restaurant: Impossible* and wondered how I got so stubborn, you now know I probably have my old man to thank.

When I was 8, we moved to Salisbury, Wiltshire, and I attended the Avon Middle School. It was about two miles away from home and I walked there every day—down a hill so steep you had to take short, stilted steps the whole way or risk tumbling down. Incidentally, this was the start of my love for sports and physical activity of all kinds, because once I got to school, this same hill was the one we'd sprint up during PT. I could just as easily have grown to hate it, but thankfully I got hooked on the runner's high.

Eventually, I got into running cross-country. I seemed to be pretty good at it; I was a very skinny, wiry kid, with decent endurance. I didn't realize at the time, though, how much my diet was holding me back— and not just in athletics, but in overall development. I'm not exaggerating when I say my diet was atrocious: I'd eat two boxes of Corn Flakes every single day, which accounted for roughly 90 percent of my calories. Now, I'm not placing all the blame on my mum, but her cooking did have something to do with it. It simply did not agree with me... Some of it was downright bad. Okay, it sucked. I'm so sorry, Mum, but you know it's true! However my talent for cooking developed, I can assure you it wasn't genetic!

The Corn Flake diet lasted from the ages of 8 to 15. During that time, I met a man who would have a profoundly positive impact on my life: David Rogers, an enormous, imposing Welshman who was my physical education teacher and taught me proper form in various exercises. Not only that, he was also my shop teacher, who helped me learn technical

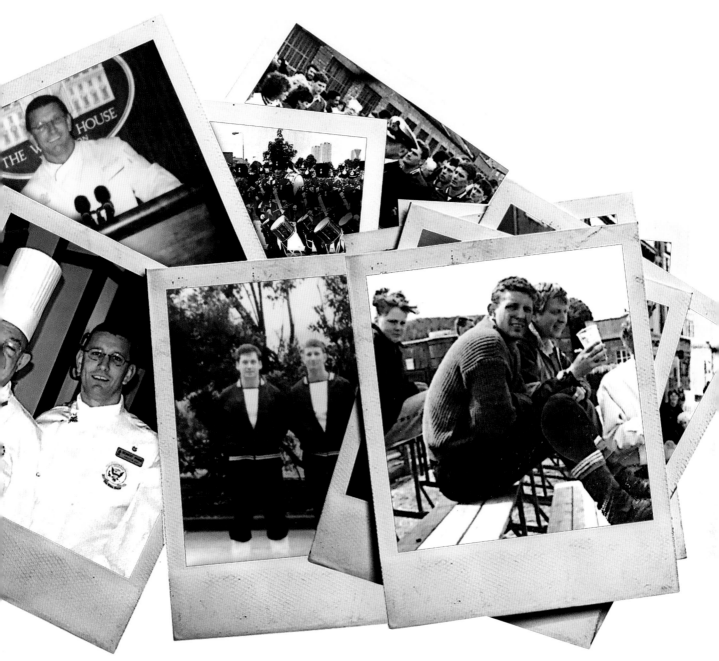

Growing up in Manchester, my family didn't have much, but that didn't stop me from dreaming big, crazy dreams. Chasing those dreams opened every good door in my life.

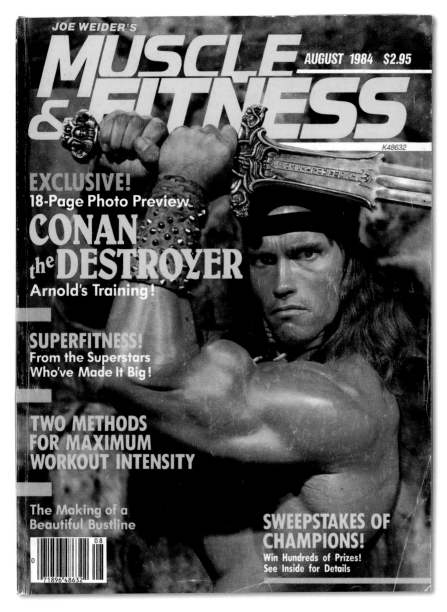

JOE WEIDER'S

MUSCLE & FITNESS

AUGUST 1984 $2.95

K48632

EXCLUSIVE!
18-Page Photo Preview
CONAN
the **DESTROYER**
Arnold's Training!

SUPERFITNESS!
From the Superstars
Who've Made It Big!

**TWO METHODS
FOR MAXIMUM
WORKOUT INTENSITY**

The Making of a
Beautiful Bustline

**SWEEPSTAKES OF
CHAMPIONS!**
Win Hundreds of Prizes!
See Inside for Details

08
0 71896 48632

> It didn't matter that I never became a bodybuilder like Arnold Schwarzenegger. So many good things in my life came from emulating him.

what might have been just a casual gesture of kindness for him, wound up changing my life: He handed me an old copy of *Muscle & Fitness* magazine.

I went home with the magazine held up high and said to my mum and dad, "Oh, look what I've got!" They nodded politely, not knowing what the hell I wanted to do with it. We didn't have any weights, and it wasn't like there was a local gym in our town back then, either. Even so, I pored over the pages and let it all soak in. I was awed by Arnold Schwarzenegger, wanting desperately to look like him and all the other guys in the magazine.

There I was, 11 years old, scrawny as hell, not eating much besides Corn Flakes, and thinking I'd look like these huge bodybuilders one day. It was beyond crazy. It was delusional.

So I don't blame my parents for wanting to write it off at first, hoping it would turn out to be just a passing phase. Every boy's fantasy is to look like Arnold Schwarzenegger, no matter how unrealistic that might be. But the more time I spent with the magazine, the more the fantasy took root. Before long, they couldn't ignore it as a passing fancy, because they had a full-blown stubborn kid on their hands, who was, naturally, begging for the Weider weight set he saw advertised in the magazine.

My parents, though, were not affluent. Dad was a painter and Mum was the manager of a home improvement store. There was no bank account full of savings for a rainy day. I didn't even have a bike. And my clothes—my mother would buy them at the secondhand store for my brother, Gary, then I'd get them when he grew out of them, meaning they were thirdhand by that point. That's how we lived. So, when faced with my demand for a weight set—the need for which they didn't really understand—Mum and Dad gave me their stock answer: "We'll try."

In the meantime, back at school, Mr. Rogers would take us through workouts. He also helped out some older, bigger rugby players

skills like woodworking and metalwork.

One day at the start of woodworking class, Mr. Rogers lumbered up to me, squinted his eyes, sized me up, and said, "You should be playing rugby, boy-o!" Mind you, I was a shy kid, and had just gotten the hang of playing football (or soccer, as Yanks call it) and was okay at it. I wasn't great, but still good enough to be on the school team, so I was hesitant to try something different. I gave Mr. Rogers a sheepish, "Maybe," but he wasn't the type of guy you ever wanted to disappoint. Deep down, I knew he'd get me to step out on a rugby pitch at some stage.

FROM CORN FLAKES TO RED MEAT: SCHWARZENEGGER, HERE I COME
Before I could play any heavy contact sports, though, I knew I needed some more meat on my bones. When I was 11, I joined the Sea Cadets, which is something like the Boy Scouts, with the difference being that the adult leaders more or less treat you like junior sailors—you go to Marine bases and onto warships, physically training as if you were joining the Royal Navy. I attacked the workouts, but again, being a bit undersized was holding me back. One of the Marines (a cook, ironically) noticed this and, in

after school, and would let me in on occasion so I could get a taste of real training. I'll never forget the clang of the iron and the feel of the bar in my hands. It was intoxicating and liberating, the best opportunity I'd had yet to improve myself. In general, I was a happy kid, but my parents took notice when I started coming home with more confidence and energy, seemingly ready to take on the world.

One day my mum found a classified ad in the paper for a used set of the Weider weights—the classic set with the gold plates—and when I got home, they were waiting for me. I'll never forget how out-of-my-mind elated I was. It was better than Ralphie finally getting the Red Ryder BB gun at the end of *A Christmas Story*. I screamed, "Are you kidding me?!"

After that, my tenacity and stubbornness took on a life of their own. Throughout the day at school, I'd daydream about going home and lifting those weights the way other kids would daydream about playing with their toys.

When I finally would get home, I'd set the weights up on our patio, flop open a copy of *Muscle & Fitness*, and get to work. While my mum cooked, she'd keep an eye on me through the kitchen window, her scrawny little boy squatting, curling, and overhead-pressing. I was mere weeks away from looking like Arnold, I just knew it!

As I got stronger and started adding muscle mass, I finally took Mr. Rogers' advice and began playing rugby. The coach made me an inside center, which, if you don't know rugby, is a position that gets a lot of carries—and takes a lot of hits. Between the weight training and hard practices, the Corn Flakes-only diet left me famished, so at long last I expanded my palate out of necessity. I started eating what the older boys told me to eat, which was, among other things, tons of red meat.

I didn't get big overnight, but I turned into a powerful kid. I was fast and could avoid hits other kids couldn't, and when I did get hit, I could shrug it off with relative ease.

While I was finally developing the way I wanted to physically, I didn't have an interest in anything at school besides phys ed and home economics. If I wasn't scheduled for one of those classes, I usually played hooky with my friends, sneaking back to my house to watch TV and lift weights. I got away with this for months, until Mum called home one day and, like a complete fool, I actually answered the phone. I can't say for sure, but that *might* be the reason why she had no issues with my joining the Royal Navy when I was barely out of puberty. (Yes, we start young in Britain.)

Eventually, the Navy would prove to be another tremendously positive experience and reinforce the pattern of my early life: When I pushed myself physically, doors began to open. I believe the same can hold true for you.

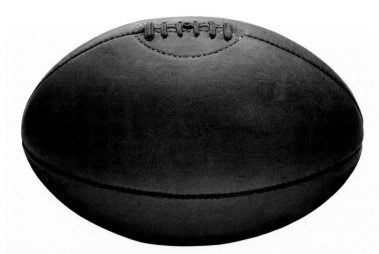

How Working Out Taught Me Not to Doubt

There is no habit more destructive than doubting oneself. For me, sports banished that doubt.

➤ Doubt, which is a manifestation of fear, will set you further from your path than missing a training session ever could. Doubting that you can and will achieve your goal removes the love of the process. Doubt will allow you to go through the motions for only so long before it finally tells you to stop because nothing will ever work—and you believe it.

"Fitness is for other people," it says, *"not for you."*

When thoughts of doubt creep into your mind, make an effort to identify them immediately. Then start the internal dialogue: Ask yourself why you feel that way and if there's a valid reason to be doubtful. Then plant the seed of the opposite thought:

I can overcome any obstacle. I will not be stopped. No matter how many setbacks I encounter, I will absolutely reach my goal.

Having a daily internal dialogue that ends on a positive note is essential to the development of the good habits that will keep you on track and ultimately bring you to your goal.

When Mr. Rogers asked me to play rugby, I doubted that I could—I didn't think I was big enough. But I started lifting weights, and in time crushed the mental opponent that was planting the seeds of doubt. When I finally started playing a few years later, I took the field every time with a single thought repeating over and over in my head: *I am the best player on this field.*

Was it true? No. Years later, I can objectively say that. But my affirmation that I *was* the best player on the field allowed me to play like I really was; it pushed me to the apex of my abilities. If I hadn't had that positive affirmation running on a loop inside my brain, there's no telling how poorly my rugby experience might have gone. I probably would have played like the kid I really was—tough and growing, yet still undersized—and eventually faded to the back as the more naturally gifted players took the spotlight.

Give yourself the same type of positive affirmation. Tell yourself that no one is going to outwork you today. Nothing anyone says can deter you. If you can't reconcile those thoughts with what you see in the mirror, remind yourself that you are still in the process of becoming the best version of you that you can possibly muster.

If you love where you're at now, while acknowledging your dissatisfaction, then the reward of getting to a better place physically and mentally is that much sweeter in the end. The naturally fit, healthy people who look great all the time can keep their genetics—what fun is that? You've been to a darker place, so you'll know how to better appreciate the light.

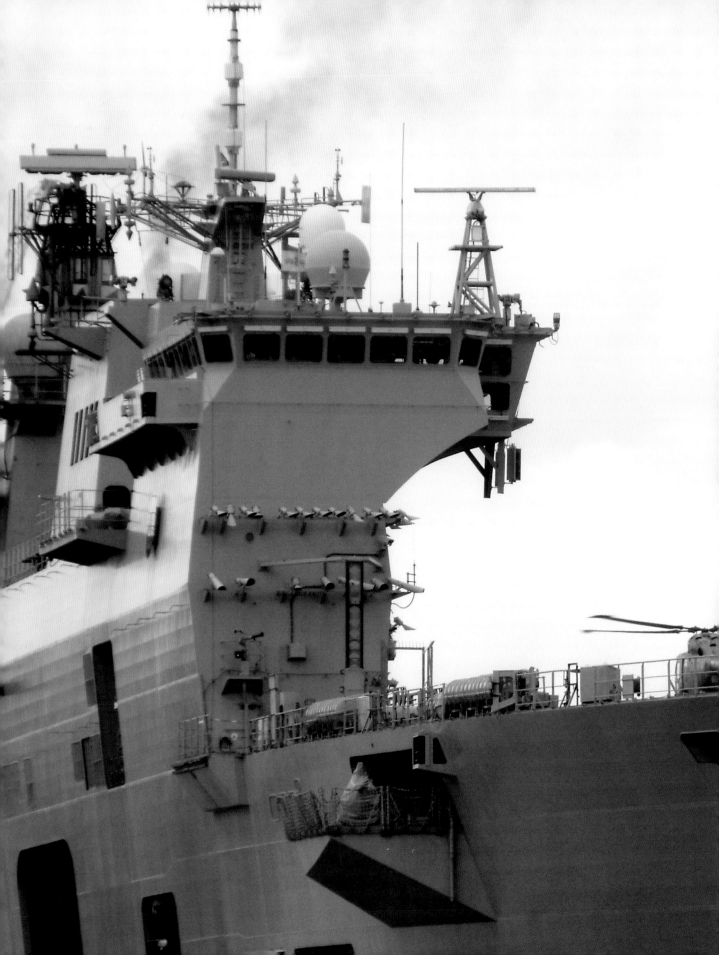

Rocking the Navy Life
(or So I Thought...)

DURING MY FIRST SIX WEEKS of training in the British Royal Navy, I flew through every PT session and obstacle course, burying the other new recruits. I owed all of that to sports and weight training. Plus, my uniforms were always judged "perfect" because, with both of my parents working as I grew up, I'd been doing my own laundry and ironing for years, and had become an expert. Now I figured I was the star recruit, continually impressing the section chief.

It turned out my performance was actually having the exact opposite effect.

One day he took me aside and said, "Listen, I'm going to throw you out of the Navy."

I was beyond shell-shocked. "Why?!" I begged. "I'm doing great, aren't I? My grades are great, my fitness is great, my uniforms are perfect."

He said, "Yes, but you're an *island*, Robert. We work in teams around here. Use some of that energy to help your classmates."

At this point I didn't yet really know how to cook, so I pitched in the best way I could: hunching over an ironing board until two in the morning, squaring away the uniforms for all 12 of my classmates. As I ironed, I instructed my team on how to do what I was doing so we'd never fail an inspection. As we finished up basic training, I came into my own and proved I wasn't just in it for myself, but was a valuable team contributor.

COOKING MY WAY UP THE LADDER

Once basic was finished, I was accepted into cook training, and surprisingly—since the talent didn't necessarily run in the family (sorry again, Mum)—established myself as a natural in the kitchen.

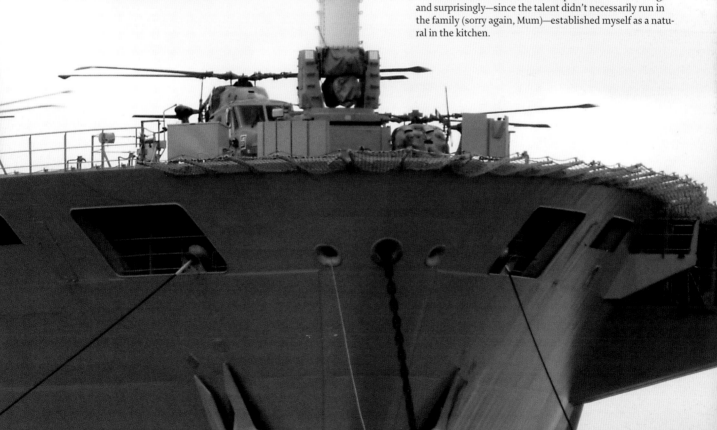

I was assigned to my first land base, HMS Pembroke, which was also the home of the Royal Navy Cookery School. I was there for about nine months, working in the main kitchen and learning everything I needed to know about not just cooking, but also the logistics of running a kitchen.

I kept lifting, taking advantage of a Navy policy called "make amends," because it gave everyone an opportunity to work out their frustrations, either by themselves or with others. As long as you were going to the gym or doing another physical activity, you could leave school an hour early. I'd lift or play soccer. Best of all, the soccer pitch gave no favor to rank. Out there we were all equals. A man could outrank you a minute before the game started and the minute it ended, but if you wanted to square him up and knock him on his ass during the game, he couldn't do a damn thing about it.

Ask the warrant officers who always seemed to have it out for me during the week: They can tell you I made the most of the policy.

WHEN I CARRIED A CANNON WHEEL FOR THE ROYAL NAVY

By the time I was assigned to the Royal Naval Air Station Culdrose, in Cornwall, I was working in a wardroom galley—an officers' dining facility—looking after 250 officers.

There, I hit the weights every day, and started to get pretty big. I also regularly ran around the base with my training partner. I loved training so much that if I hadn't already put in so much time training as a cook, I'd have asked for a transfer to become a PT instructor.

In time I was selected for the greatest honor of my naval career: I was made a wheelman in the Royal Navy Field Gun Competition. For the uninitiated, the Field Gun Competition started in 1907 as a way for sailors to prove their worth by moving a cannon, in pieces, as fast as possible over varied terrain and challenging obstacles. Eighteen men would work in tandem to hoist a ton and a half of equipment over an obstacle course three times the length of a football field—in under three minutes. It was a grueling test of strength and cardiovascular endurance, similar to a World's Strongest Man contest but with coordination between team members being a major factor.

My job as a wheelman, as you might have guessed, was to carry one of the cannon's wheels, an unwieldy 120-pound piece of equipment. If you're not familiar with the competition, I'd encourage you to look it up on YouTube—it's a truly fascinating spectacle.

The training for the Field Gun Competition was more grueling than the competition itself. My team would wake up at five o'clock in the morning and go for a run, two groups of 20 men running in formation around Whale

+ **WHAT FUELS ME**

Right: Taking part in the Royal Navy's Field Gun Competition was the most grueling athletic endeavor I've ever experienced.

Far right: With my wife, Gail, who taught me to eat healthier than I ever had before.

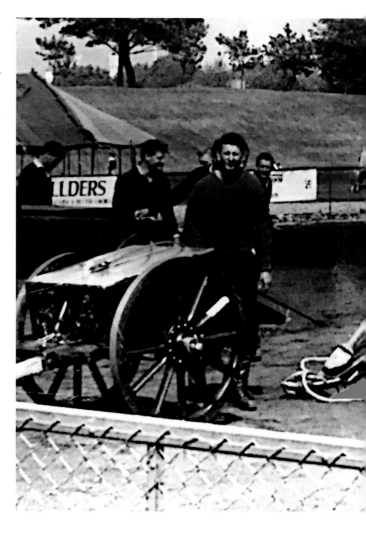

Island, an old gunnery school. We'd finish by doing pyramid circuits; you start with a high number of reps on any exercise, like pushups, work your way down to a smaller number, then work your way back to the highest number. For example, doing sets of 40, 30, 20, 10, 20, 30, 40, in that order. Those are some of the most intense workouts I've ever done.

When we got back, we'd shower, change, and eat. None of us was small, all of us were still growing, and we were working as hard as we ever had. The appetite we worked up was so tremendous we'd each eat a dozen eggs for breakfast. We tried to keep protein high and stay relatively healthy, but in truth we were eating whatever we wanted. At the time it was fine, but it created a problem I'd have to deal with some years later.

I'm sad to say the Field Gun Competition ended in 1999; budget cuts and the extremely dangerous nature of the event (a competitor died in 1982 after being struck by a swinging log) conspired to bring about its demise. Nevertheless, taking part in it remains one of the proudest moments of my life.

MY HEALTH WAS A CASUALTY OF MY SUCCESS

After I left the military I worked a number of jobs, most notably as an executive chef on a cruise ship and at Donald Trump's Taj Mahal Casino Hotel. Being able to create gourmet meals for a huge number of people ideally suited me for my first show on Food Network, *Dinner: Impossible,* where they'd drop me blind into a brand-new situation every week and I'd be forced to whip up something amazing for a few hundred people in just a couple of hours.

My career took off to a degree I had never imagined. By the time I met my wife Gail—a dynamic and stunningly beautiful professional wrestler—in 2008, I was training hard, but still eating like a 20-year-old. My thinking was: *I work my ass off all day and train my ass off at night. What I eat doesn't matter.* So I ate anything I wanted, with fried food being a major pitfall. I love fish and chips, pizza, burgers, pasta. I ate some *amazing* variations of these foods, but in terms of the macronu-

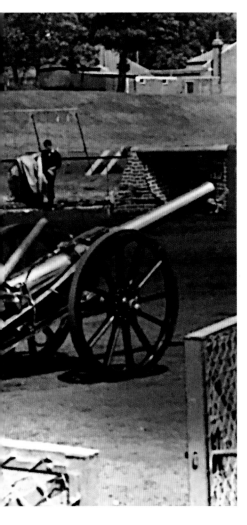

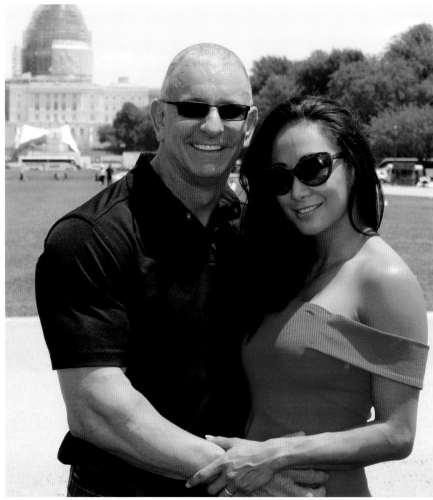

trients I was getting—and the micronutrients these foods lacked—it wasn't much better than eating regular fast food.

As most ex-athletes learn, the eating habits you develop when you're playing competitively don't serve you well in the years that follow, as activity levels decline and the metabolism slows. A lot of ex-ruggers and footballers get fat. Others, like me, show few outward signs of ailment, but suffer on the inside.

I didn't gain a huge amount of weight, but all those years of eating whatever the hell I wanted, not getting enough sleep, and thinking that getting to the gym would bail me out finally caught up with me when my doctor told me I had high cholesterol and high blood pressure, and put me on several medications. I was just another statistic, one of the world's 330 million people diagnosed with high blood pressure and 147 million with high cholesterol. Factor in my stress level and lack of sleep, and I was a ticking time bomb—a heart attack waiting to happen.

When Gail got to know me and learned

about the medications I was taking, she was shocked. How could this guy who looked healthy, lifted weights, and cooked for a living not have his health in order? Why wasn't he cooking better meals for himself, and making his health a priority?

In my mind, the proof this didn't matter was in my physique. I was muscular, relatively lean, and athletic. Oftentimes one's physique and health mirror each another; but in my case, they didn't. Moreover, the medication only put a Band-Aid on the problem.

It was Gail who taught me that training is only about 20 percent of the battle. The other 80 percent? That part takes place entirely within the kitchen. Here I was, a trained professional chef with all the weapons I needed to win that battle—and I didn't even know it.

Gail did all the right things out of necessity. The world in which she makes her living isn't kind to a woman who loses her figure; plus, it would be impossible for her to remain athletic if she didn't have an impeccable diet. Regardless of your opinion of pro wrestling, there's

no denying how hard these men and women work, getting into the ring almost every single night and handling a brutal travel schedule. Gail's been able to do it for years in absolutely phenomenal shape. She owes a big part of it to her training regimen—and an even bigger part of it to her diet.

She taught me about things like always keeping healthy meals and snacks at the ready. But more than that, she inspired me to change, to take better care of myself and use my culinary skills to make healthy meals that didn't sacrifice what I love so much about food: the taste. I tinkered for several years to strike the perfect balance, to create the recipes now before you in this book. Combine them with the training plan—which I've followed myself for nearly two decades—and you have all the tools you need to reshape your life.

I'm excited to share these experiences with you, and quite frankly honored that you've welcomed them into your life. The overarching lesson here is that if I can change, then you can change.

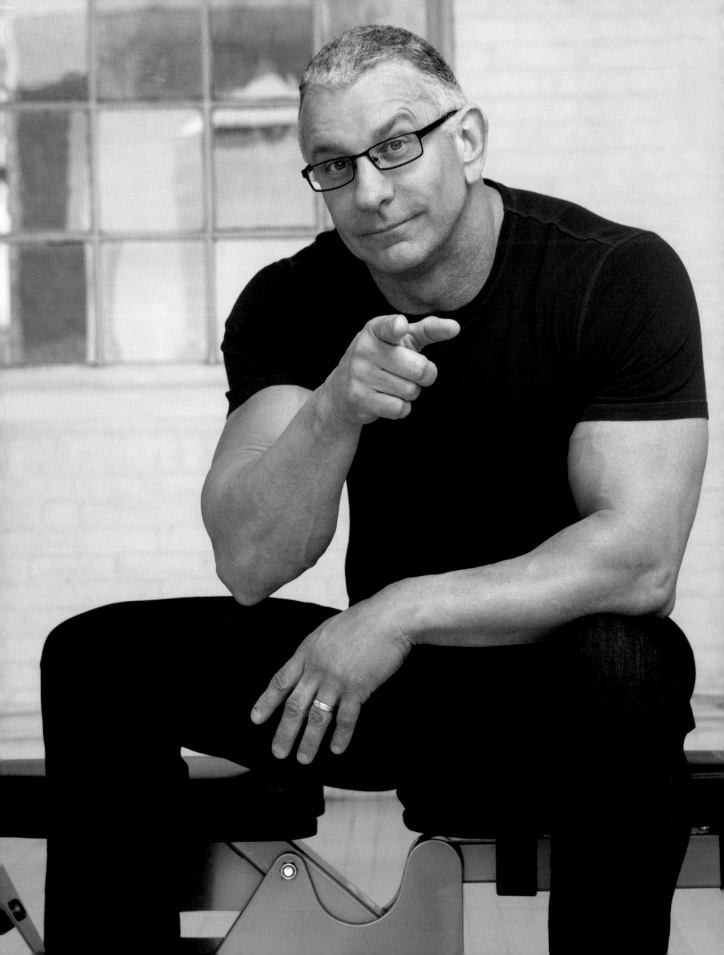

Why You'll Make It Stick This Time

WE ALL FALL OFF THE WAGON. I've done it. You've done it. Arnold Schwarzenegger has done it. How long you choose to stay down directly impacts your quality of life. Let's say you move, change jobs, or start a family. Pick any number of huge, life-altering, stress-inducing major changes and usually the first things that go out the window are getting to the gym and eating healthy meals. This is normal.

> Failure happens, but you need to be honest about why you failed. Don't blame external factors.

But you have to learn to recognize when it's happening and pull yourself out of the rut before time slips away from you. Here's why it will work this time.

THIS TIME YOU'LL USE MOMENTUM TO YOUR ADVANTAGE

A week away from the gym can so easily become a month, then two, and before you know it a whole year or more of your life has gone by. It happens because there is momentum to all of our actions. Activity begets more activity. Laziness begets more laziness. The hardest part of any physical transformation is the initial attempt to shift that momentum away from laziness and into activity. It can take from three to nine weeks (probably closer to nine!) of consistent effort to form a habit—for example, getting to the point at which it becomes normal and effortless to get up and go to the gym before work—and only a week away to kill the habit. Once you get past that three-week mark, it is absolutely essential to stay the course. But, lucky for you, it also starts to feel more natural.

One thing I can't identify with is the frustration people have when they're a month into a new fitness and healthy eating plan, and they say they're not making progress fast enough. Think of it this way: How long have you been doing nothing and eating like crap? A year? Five years? Ten or more? Think about how long you've been doing things the wrong way before you complain about how long it's taking to right the ship.

No, it shouldn't be a straight 1:1 trade-off—if you've been doing nothing for five years, it shouldn't take you five years to get back in shape. But if you've done a lot of damage to yourself over a long period of time,

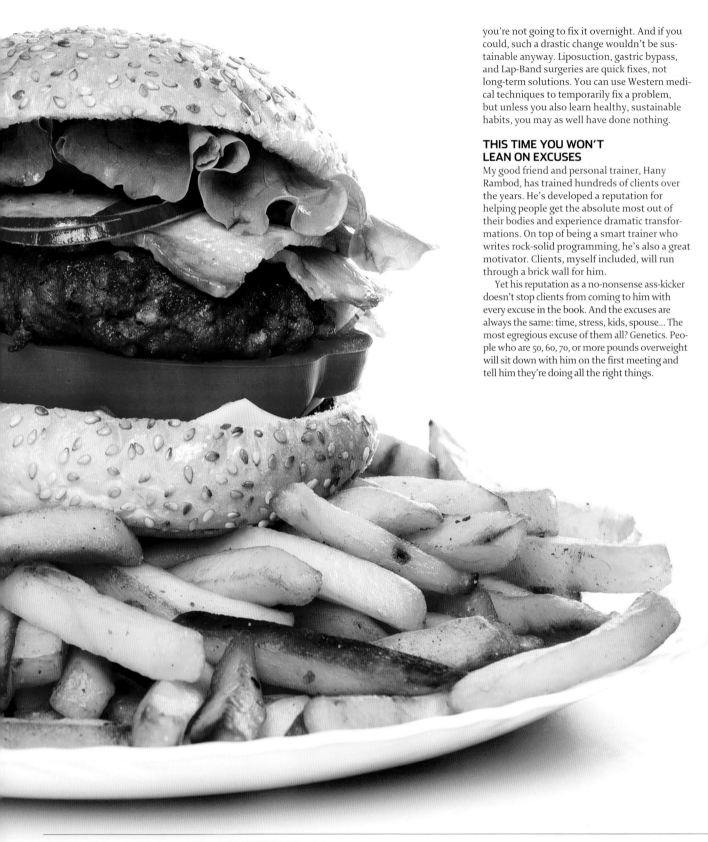

you're not going to fix it overnight. And if you could, such a drastic change wouldn't be sustainable anyway. Liposuction, gastric bypass, and Lap-Band surgeries are quick fixes, not long-term solutions. You can use Western medical techniques to temporarily fix a problem, but unless you also learn healthy, sustainable habits, you may as well have done nothing.

THIS TIME YOU WON'T LEAN ON EXCUSES

My good friend and personal trainer, Hany Rambod, has trained hundreds of clients over the years. He's developed a reputation for helping people get the absolute most out of their bodies and experience dramatic transformations. On top of being a smart trainer who writes rock-solid programming, he's also a great motivator. Clients, myself included, will run through a brick wall for him.

Yet his reputation as a no-nonsense ass-kicker doesn't stop clients from coming to him with every excuse in the book. And the excuses are always the same: time, stress, kids, spouse... The most egregious excuse of them all? Genetics. People who are 50, 60, 70, or more pounds overweight will sit down with him on the first meeting and tell him they're doing all the right things.

"But I do eat well!"

"I work out five days a week!"

"I don't eat junk food."

And then...

"I think I just have a slow metabolism."

In essence, they're saying it's impossible for them to get in shape. They looked up some disorder on Wikipedia and convinced themselves they're part of an infinitesimally small segment of the population who are predisposed to being obese no matter what they eat. They'd rather assume they have an extreme glandular disorder that affects a very small number of people than put in the work necessary to change.

If they really think that, why work out at all? They might as well just kick back, turn on the TV, and pass the Doritos.

I can't stand this excuse. Hany can't either. On its surface it seems like a harmless dodge: Here's someone who's tried a dozen different diets and workouts but never gotten the desired results. So, the thinking goes, "It must be genetic. It must be my metabolism."

But if you look deeper into this excuse, it's far more sinister. It allows you to disavow all personal responsibility. Further, it assumes that all previous attempts at getting in shape were *perfect* attempts that gave all parts of the training and diet plan enough time to produce results. And what, exactly, is enough time to determine if a program is working?

Well, how long was it, you said, that you've been eating like crap? Then you go on a diet for a few weeks and expect to have rippling muscles and six-pack abs?

When it's put like that, do you see how ludicrous an excuse that is?

I ran into the same problem on countless occasions while filming *Restaurant: Impossible*. I'd come across restaurant owners who were $100,000 in debt, their food sucked, their kitchen was filthy, their décor was depressing, and they had no customers. I'd come in, pinpoint where they were wasting money, why their food tasted awful, and why half the staff deserved to be fired. Without fail they'd tell me, "But I do the right things! I'm very careful about my menu, I think the food tastes good, and my staff isn't that bad!"

"Then why are you in debt?" I'd ask.

Now ask yourself the same question about your physique and your health. You think you eat healthy. You think you train hard. You think you do the right things.

Then why are you still fat?

Don't bother thinking of an answer. I've got it here: You don't work nearly as hard as you think you do, and you don't eat well on a consistent enough basis. Your body represents the sum total of what you do *most* of the time, not some of the time. The universe is very fair in that sense: What you get out of things equals what you put into them. Your body is no different. You're no different.

Stop thinking you are, then progress can begin.

THIS TIME YOU'LL ENJOY WHAT YOU EAT

I started writing a monthly food column for *Muscle & Fitness* magazine back in March of 2011. It was a natural collaboration: The healthy chef delivers a healthy recipe every month. Done. Plus, as I said, I'd read the magazine as a kid—it was really my first training partner. Joe Weider's principles became the basis for how I'd train for the rest of my life. *M&F* has a well-earned reputation as "the Iron Bible."

2011 was also the perfect time for a collaboration. It's a different era now, of course, but back in the '80s, the nutrition content of *M&F* and other magazines in the category was, to be kind, lacking. It taught people how to eat like competitors, which is to say, measure every last gram of protein, fat, and carbs they put into their bodies at every meal—but do nothing to flavor the food. It was grilled chicken, lean red meat, plain vegetables, rice, and very little besides that.

Many fitness enthusiasts, especially competitors, still eat like this today. But thankfully, more and more people are learning it doesn't have to be this way. You can prep and add sophisticated flavors to your food without making it unhealthy. You can eat like a foodie, have delicious, satisfying meals, and never stray from your goals.

Okay, maybe you don't identify yourself as a foodie, and maybe you couldn't care less about cooking anything close to a "gourmet" meal. Fair enough. Feel free to close the book and go eat plain grilled chicken and broccoli. But before you do, know this: That strategy works only for a handful of people who are both 1) extremely dedicated and used to eating that way, and 2) naturally less susceptible to cravings.

I've met some people who possess this combination of qualities, but I'm not one of them, and I never will be. I eat for flavor and satisfaction. Granted, I'm generally disciplined enough to eat only when I'm hungry—not when I get bored or upset—but when I eat I want to eat well. Hence my choice of profession.

THIS TIME YOU'LL UNDERSTAND WHAT YOU'RE DOING

So far I've shared the parts of my story that are most pertinent for the task ahead of you. I've shared how I had an early interest in physical fitness and in cooking. Now, you might not be able to identify with these specific aspects of my life, but don't dismiss my story because yours is different. The path I traveled to where I am today might look different from your own, but breaking my bad habits was just as difficult and painful for me as you believe it will be for you. I need you to know about this part of my life because, at its base level, it really isn't very different from what most people go through.

Despite my early interest in sports, I never really did more than dabble—doing just enough to stay in respectable shape until I was forced to take things seriously.

That same interest in sports caused wear and tear on my body that eventually broke me down. I had a total hip replacement in 2013. Yet, to my absolute shock, my full recovery took less than two months. After that I was back in the gym, squatting and deadlifting with decent weight. Most people didn't even know I had undergone surgery. I owe my recovery entirely to having cleaned up my diet and gotten serious about my gym regimen when I was faced with the consequences of high blood pressure and cholesterol.

So I understand the struggle you have. I know there are things you'd rather do than concentrate on your health. I hope you can look at my story and see shades of what you've gone through. I hope you can look at it and see that it's possible to change.

Understand this: Most often, fitness regimens fail because the people undertaking them don't truly believe they're worthy of the result. It's easy to look at someone who's superfit and healthy and place him or her on a pedestal. Fitness magazines do this all time, albeit unintentionally, because for every reader who's inspired by the cover model and wants to learn more about the habits that can effect such a change, there are many more people who are turned in the opposite direction. The images can seem too perfect, so readers walk away in disbelief and further entrench their minds in the notion that health and fitness are for other people, not for them.

Deep down you might have these ideas yourself and not even know it. So here's a test: Flip to the picture of me with my shirt off on page 35, then turn back here. Now: When you saw the picture and noticed the six-pack abs, did you say to yourself, "I want to be just as fit as he is when I'm his age!" Or did you say, "God, this guy's a nut!" Which way do you lean between those two responses? Am I nuts? Or do I just care deeply about my health? Is my state of fitness achievable for everyone, or am I just another fanatic, putting on a show?

If you lean toward incredulous, then we've identified the biggest part of your problem. Despite protests to the contrary, I'm really not in "outrageous" shape for my age. What I have done, however, is tap into my full potential.

You have the same potential within you if you'd only have the courage to accept it. I say "courage" because, once you've acknowledged

> The way you look now isn't the result of genetics, the way you were raised, your tough job, or the crazy kids who take up all your time. You look this way because of what you've put into your body, and the exercise you've chosen—or chosen *not*—to do.

that you too can have this, then the onus is on you to do something about it. That's why most people never make it past the initial step of deciding to get in shape.

Breaking this mental barrier is more important and harder to do than any workout or any diet. This is the fulcrum upon which all your success hinges. If you really can't get yourself to believe in your own considerable potential and your ability to absolutely achieve a high level of fitness—and happiness—in your life, then there's nothing I can do for you.

This is your war, the first battle of which will be waged entirely inside your own head. Affirm yourself daily. Tell yourself that you can and will do this. Wake up in the morning, splash cold water on your face, and stare deeply into the black pupils looking back at you from the mirror. What do you see inside the black? It just goes on forever, doesn't it? There's no better metaphor for your own potential.

Now find your "why"—as in, Why do this? My "why" was a deep desire to be around a long time for my kids and my wife, to continue my career at a high level and go on providing for them. Is your own "why" so different? Don't you want to feel good as you walk through life—all the time, not just some of the time? Put yourself and your family at the top of your list of priorities. You deserve not to feel self-conscious as you walk down the street or lie on the beach. You shouldn't have to stockpile a flattering wardrobe to hide what you hate about your body.

You deserve to be your healthiest and fittest self—and your family deserves that, too.

THIS TIME YOU WON'T BE DOING IT ALONE

From the start, I enjoyed sports, but didn't know how to eat. I liked my life in the Navy but didn't know how to be a team player. I landed a terrific career, but was still unhealthy because I hadn't mastered all aspects of being fit—and didn't have a pressing reason to do so.

The lessons of each phase of my life speak to the basic need for a life in balance. My love of athletics and cooking weren't enough to make me healthy. Getting diagnosed with high blood pressure and high cholesterol wasn't enough to snap me out of bad habits. Just as I'd done early on in my naval career, I was working alone, failing to realize that a great team could take me so much further than I could ever go by myself. Years of playing sports and taking part in the Field Gun Competition should have taught me the value of teamwork, yet I saw them as only isolated athletic events, not something I could carry over into everyday life.

Lo and behold, Gail turned out to be the best teammate a man could ever ask for. A wake-up call from her set me on the right path. And

when I started eating healthy, all my blood pressure and cholesterol medications found their way into the trash can.

Who are your teammates—your husband, wife, kids, brothers, sisters, friends? I want you to use them as your support group as you undertake this change. Tell them what you're trying to do and why. Tell them you need their encouragement to reinforce the bold new decisions you're making.

If there's anyone close to you in your life who won't do this—who encourages you to continue with the same old poor habits that made you unhappy and unhealthy—you need to reevaluate your relationship with that person. Like a diet of straight fast food, some of the people in our lives can be toxic. Have the courage to momentarily step outside yourself and look at the situation objectively. You can only get so far without love and support. To reach my ultimate goal and start living up to my full potential, I needed at least one great teammate. I know the same goes for you.

THIS TIME YOU'LL BE COMPLETELY HONEST WITH YOURSELF

I want you to go to a room where you'll have privacy and a mirror. Bathroom, bedroom, doesn't matter as long as it's quiet—no TV, no phones, nobody to break your concentration. You need a moment alone with yourself. Just get in there, close the door, and stand in front of the mirror.

Now I want you to take your clothes off. Everything. Try not to imagine the sound of my voice telling you to do this, because you'll either burst out laughing or never watch my shows again! But I still need you to do it because it's important.

First, have a long look in the mirror and take it all in. Look at yourself from head to toe. Look at your face, your neck, your shoulders and arms. Look at your chest, your stomach, your legs and feet. Don't suck in your gut. Don't flex your arms. Relax and just be. No one else is there to judge you.

Next, turn sideways and get a look at your profile. Then turn the other way. Look yourself up and down. If you have a hand mirror now

would be a good time to use it, because a look at your backside wouldn't hurt, either. I need you to take full stock of yourself right now. Look at everything that's going on with your body.

It's time to ask yourself a question: Am I happy with this?

What's your answer? Do you like the way you look? Would you be embarrassed for other people to see you this way? Or proud?

If you haven't been hitting the gym and eating healthy food on a consistent basis, then I doubt you like the way you look.

For most people, the mirror self-examination is an incredibly tough exercise, because even though we "see" ourselves in the mirror each morning, we tend to be very careful about how we do it. We subconsciously suck in that gut, stand up a little straighter than normal, or flex muscles that are relaxed most of the day.

We do this partly out of vanity and partly out of the need to get through our days with at least a modicum of confidence. None of us wants to step out into the world without feeling good about ourselves, so in the mirror we pull in our stomachs and stand erect. We do this so often we lose sight of what it is we really look like when we're in our natural state—standing with normal posture, all muscles relaxed.

Now, here's the second part of this exercise, and it's just as vital that you follow through with it: Whatever it was you saw in your reflection, take ownership of it.

Accept that the way you look now isn't the result of genetics, the way you were raised, your tough job, or the crazy kids who take up all your time. You look this way because of what you've put into your body and the exercise you've chosen—or chosen *not*—to do.

There are no mitigating factors. Taking ownership of how you look and feel now is absolutely essential; having power over what you've done to yourself gives you absolute power to change yourself. It's that simple.

Now take one last look in the mirror, and say, "I alone did this. And I can change it—starting right now."

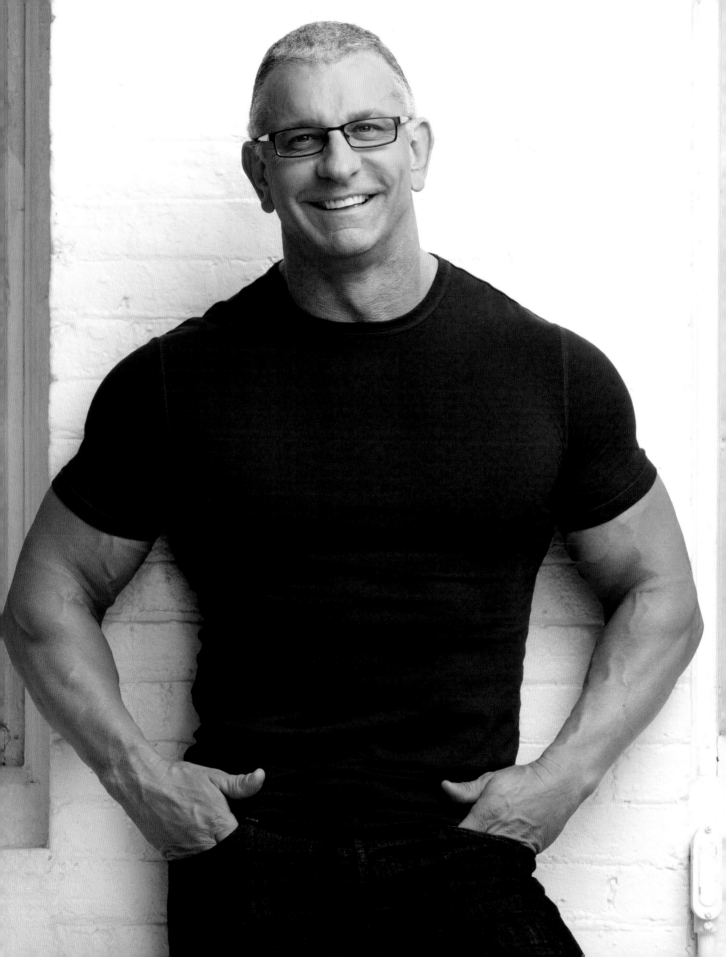

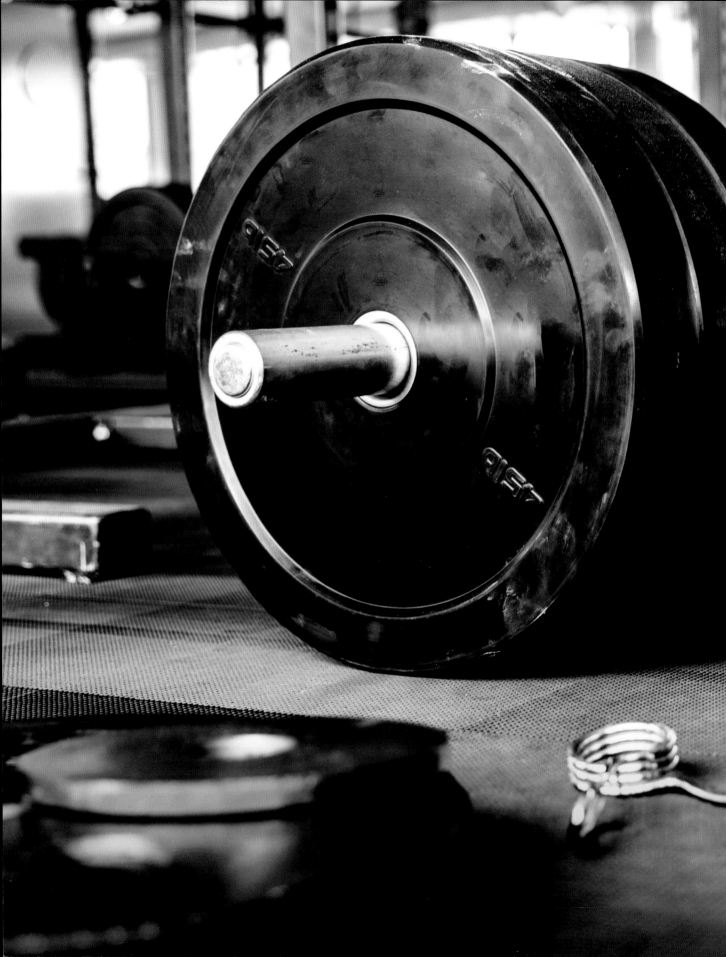

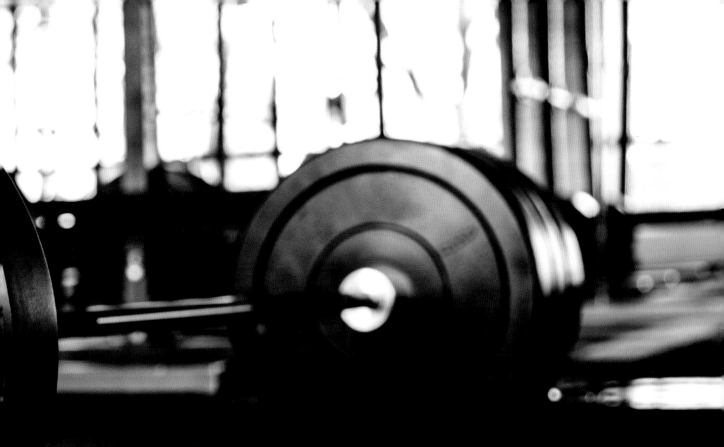

No-Excuses
Training
Success tactics that get results

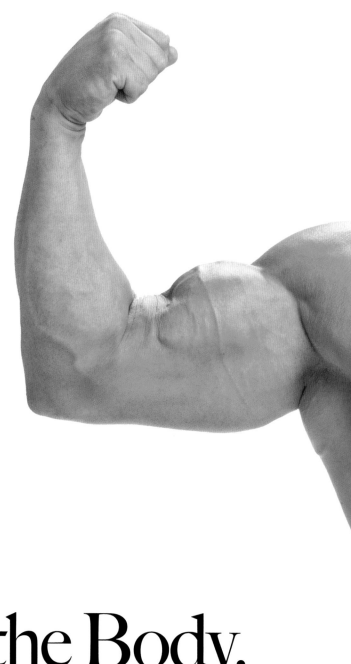

In order to flourish, life demands balance. The mind follows the body, and the body follows the mind. I know intellectuals with genius-level smarts who, despite all their knowledge, neglect their bodies. As bright as they are, their paths are limited.

Conversely, I know too many athletically gifted men and women who, sadly, decided early on they wouldn't bother with their studies, but would rely instead on wherever their "great genes" could take them. They learned the hard way that, even for exceptional athletes, the chances of turning pro and making a living that way are incredibly small. When they washed out they had nothing to fall back on.

These are extreme examples of a basic concept, and I cite them to reinforce how unwise it is to live an unbalanced life. Even if you don't fall into one of these categories, the principle still applies: If you, like so many people today, put career and money before your physical well-being, you place yourself at risk. Your spirit, mind, and body all deserve an equal amount of love and devotion from you, their caretaker. That's why the "I have no time" excuse absolutely, 100 percent does not fly.

My travel schedule is bananas, but if I can take care of my body with the innumerable time constraints I face on a daily basis, then you can, too.

The following is a field guide to getting started the right way.

The Mind Follows the Body. The Body Follows the Mind.

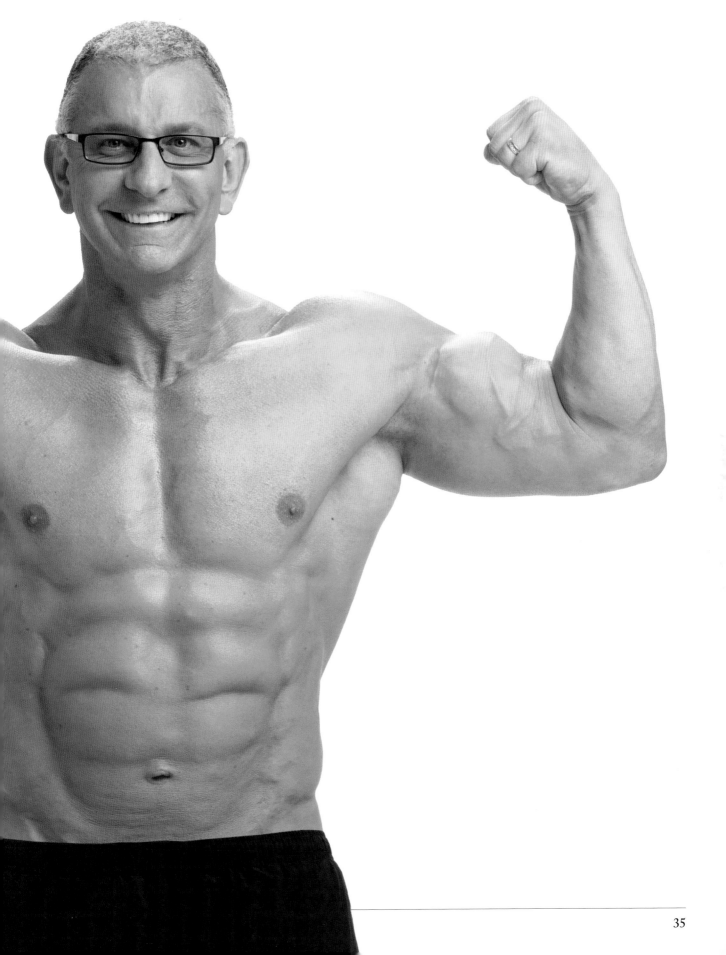

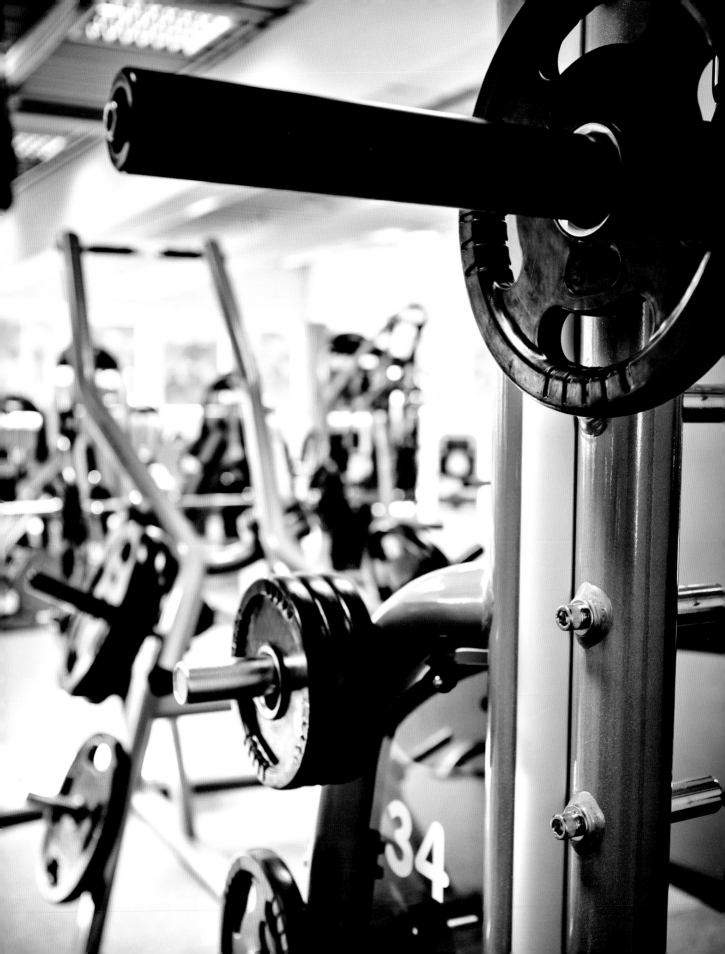

Join a Real Gym

Success Tactic No. 1

THERE'S A MYTH THAT'S BEEN PERPETUATED by big corporate chain gyms like Planet Fitness—it's the idea that simply going to the gym is a commendable act that puts you in a special league of people who are better than those who don't go at all. As with any myth, there's a grain of truth to it. I've always said you'll get results from whatever training program you pick up because something's always better than nothing.

But this kind of thinking can take you only so far; and if it's the only basis you have for staying healthy and fit, then you're bound to find yourself mired in the cycle of failure, which I'll outline for you soon.

The best analogy I can make is that people who simply have gym memberships are like diet soda drinkers who develop a false sense of security about their overall eating habits—who, because they're not drinking full-sugar soda, think they've earned special rewards in the form of fried foods, pastries, and the like. When I go into a corporate chain gym and see the number of people who do nothing more than trundle along on a treadmill and think they're doing enough for their health, I find it truly alarming.

And I've come to realize that it's not just America's fast-food lifestyle, but also a large part of its gym culture that are to blame for the current obesity epidemic.

I'm not saying it's *impossible* to get a good workout at a gym like this—I train in plenty of these facilities, especially when I'm on the road and don't have any other options. But I do think that belonging to a corporate gym makes getting fit a bit more difficult. Here's why:

At most corporate gyms...

...FEWER MEMBERS ARE MOTIVATED

You're going to be more willing to train hard if you're around other motivated people. You may not be totally comfortable with the idea of joining a gym frequented by bodybuilders and powerlifters, but in time their dedication will start to rub off on you. Since motivation is usually lacking in corporate facilities, this can put you behind the eight ball from the day you join.

...THE EQUIPMENT IS ALL WRONG

The ratio of cardio to weight-training equipment is typically out of whack. If most of the floor space is dedicated to treadmills and ellipticals, with very little space for power racks, Olympic lifting platforms, and free weights, then it's not a gym for people serious about getting fit.

...THEY WON'T LET YOU WORK HARD

Planet Fitness and some other corporate chain gyms forbid deadlifting, which is probably *the* most important functional lift. Everyone should be deadlifting, regardless of age or gender. If you're young, no single lift gives you more bang for your buck, stimulating muscle fibers in several major muscle groups. If you're older, there are few exercises that can rival the deadlift for helping increase bone density and warding off osteoporosis. I know people who have actually reversed osteopenia (the precursor to osteoporosis) merely by adding deadlifts to their program. If you walk into a gym that has a rule forbidding the deadlift—usually because the plates clanking on the ground is considered too noisy—then it's really not a gym at all.

...THEY DO "PIZZA DAY"

Or Bagel Day. Or any of the other "membership appreciation" gimmicks where management dishes out a bunch of simple carbs as treats to show how much they appreciate your business. If they really cared about you they'd learn a thing or two about nutrition and stop offering you junk food. Tootsie Rolls at the counter? This is either aggressively stupid or just flat-out mean. In either case, only a horrible gym would do this.

...THEY DON'T REALLY WANT YOU THERE

The business model of most corporate chain gyms is predicated on the fact that most of the members won't show up. If all the members *did* show up regularly, the gym would be far over capacity and become an instant fire hazard. These gyms make their money off the members who stay home, not the ones who come in and induce real wear and tear on the equipment. They can afford to make the membership very cheap because the vast majority of members paying the $10 a month will rarely see the inside.

SO... how will you know when you've found a real gym? For one thing, it probably won't cost just $10 a month. For another, it'll have at least as much weight-training equipment as cardio machines. Many more of the members will actually be in decent shape, and the front desk won't offer you pizza and bagels. Oh, and a heavy barbell might just hit the floor every now and then. Don't worry—this is the way a gym is supposed to sound.

As for chain gyms that do it the right way: Gold's Gym and World Gym are two names you can trust. Look for these near you, or scout the nearest mom-and-pop gym.

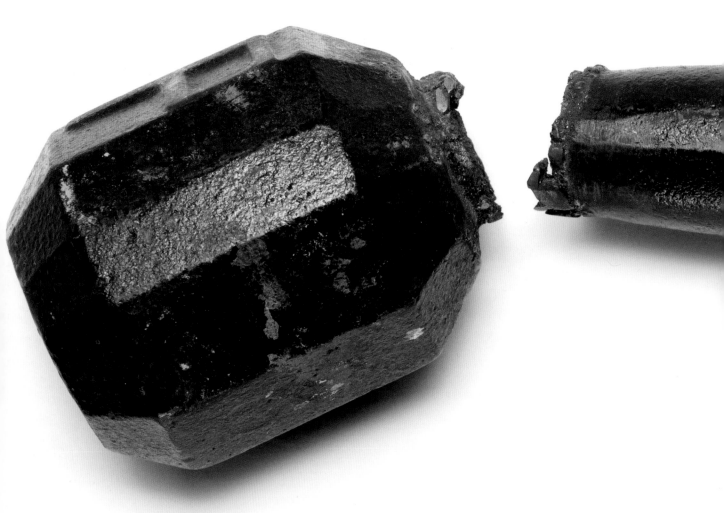

Avoid the Cycle of Fitness Failure

Success Tactic No. 2

MOST PEOPLE WHO ARE OVERWEIGHT AND OUT OF SHAPE have tried to get fit at some point. You'd have to search the world over to find someone who's never tried even a little. But the vast majority of attempts to get in shape end in failure. The people who fail usually follow this very common cycle:

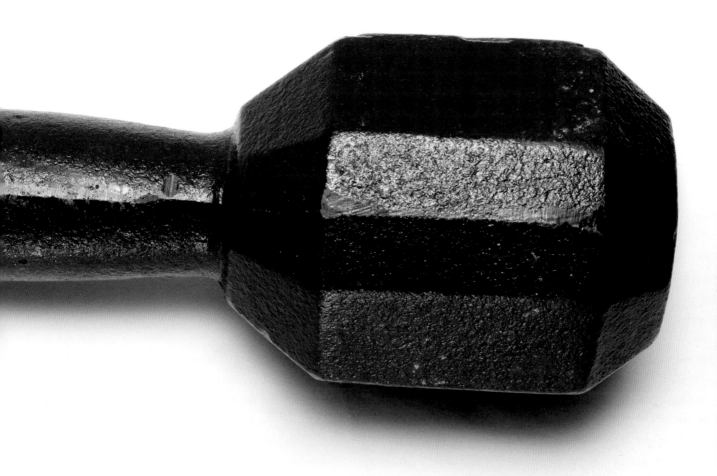

1 THEY CHANGE EVERYTHING AT ONCE

A person has a goal in mind, and resolves to do whatever it takes every day to achieve it. In fitness, this often takes the form of a complete beginner deciding to go to the gym every single day and greatly reduce calorie intake from previous norms.

2 THEY BURN OUT TOO FAST

The individual pours an excessive amount of energy into the initial efforts, which exhaust them because the plan (e.g., go to the gym every day for two hours) is too ambitious. Proper recovery time isn't allowed for either, so they quickly become even more tired and run-down. And since they haven't broken their goal into small, achievable steps they can continue to follow in a *sensible* way, enthusiasm begins to diminish.

3 THEY FAIL—THEN START OVER AGAIN THE SAME WAY

The individual meets with failure (usually in the form of a weekend eating and/or drinking binge), and the aggressive diet and training plan becomes a distant memory. Eventually, frustration reminds them of how dissatisfied they are, and brings them back to Step 1. Of course, if concrete changes haven't been made, the next go-round proves even more difficult; the wound of failure is fresh, and the idea of traveling the same road again is even more disheartening.

Be patient. Trying to make progress overnight—and constantly reevaluating your methods—leads to frustration and failure.

Does any of that sound like something you've experienced? Maybe more than once? I've seen enough people in my life go through this cycle to say for certain that it's very common.

But there's a way to beat the cycle needlessly tearing down so many well-intentioned folks. Here are some steps to follow:

TO SUCCEED INSTEAD: PUT YOUR GOALS DOWN ON PAPER

Yes, *real paper.* Go get yourself a nice notebook and pen, and write what you definitely aim to achieve. I know, most people keep notes and reminders on their phones and tablets these days, but I don't think these devices are an adequate replacement for old-fashioned pen and paper in this instance. If you write your goals down in an app or computer program, they're buried inside the memory of a device, and require you to open a program anytime you wish to see them.

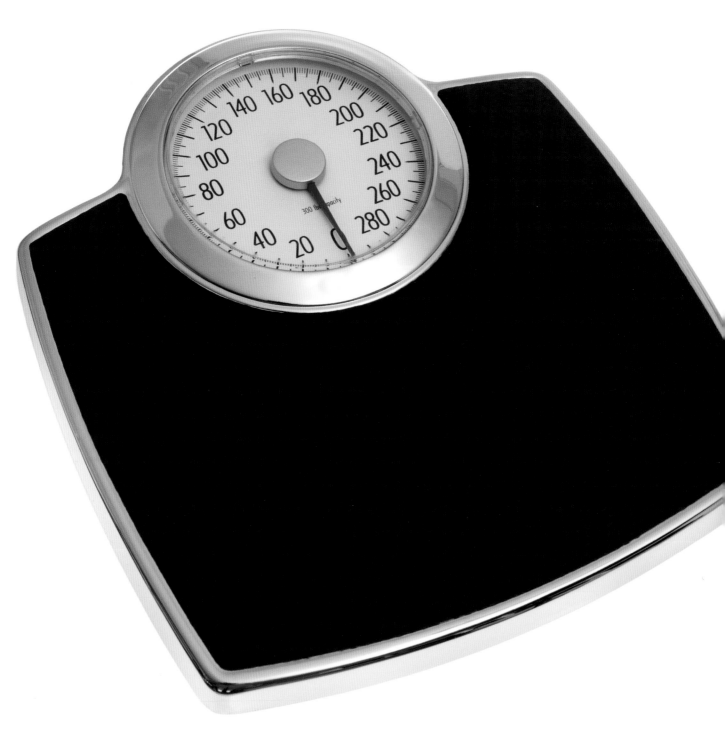

Write your goals down on paper and they take physical, concrete form and have more power to influence your daily actions—especially when you write them out several times and hang them in different places, like on the fridge, at your desk at work, and beside your bed. For a goal to grow in your mind and take the place of other useless or detrimental thoughts, it needs to be omnipresent in your life. Seeing your goal everywhere

you turn is a way to give it power it wouldn't have if it only existed in your mind or somewhere on a computer.

BE SPECIFIC

"Lose 40 pounds" is not concrete enough. "Lose 40 pounds by July 1" is better. Now, take that a step further and create a series of more modest targets to help you reach your objective.

Losing 40 pounds is an admirable goal, but to do it, you'll need to stick to losing a safe—and sustainable—maximum of three to four pounds every two weeks.

Go to the box at the top of the next page to see what a sample goal of losing 40 pounds by July 1 should look like when you write it down on January 1. You'll check off each goal once it's been achieved.

Sample Goal Checklist

I, (NAME HERE), resolve to lose 40 pounds by July 1, 20XX.

_____ *I will lose 4 pounds by January 14.*

_____ *I will lose 4 pounds by January 31.*

_____ *I will lose 4 pounds by February 14.*

_____ *I will lose 4 pounds by February 28.*

[AND SO FORTH UNTIL JULY 1]

DECIDE TO STAY FLEXIBLE

Of course, in a perfect world you'd be able to stick with that same checklist from beginning to end; but even the best-laid plans hit plateaus and encounter other unforeseen setbacks. The key is to stay on top of your list.

Do not allow a missed check mark to waylay the entire goal: Simply start again on a fresh sheet of paper with a revised list. If you leave the original list with missed deadlines in front of you, it will only serve as a reminder of your lapse, and could become a trigger for you to fall back into bad habits.

VISUALIZE YOURSELF AS HAVING ALREADY WON

To be truly successful, you can never accept defeat. You must instead look at difficulties or missteps as merely temporary setbacks. Napoleon Hill wrote about this extensively in his classic book *Think and Grow Rich,* which set the stage for the entire self-help genre as we know it, and I can't recommend it highly enough. Hill's principles of success can be applied to virtually any area of your life. As he teaches readers how to accrue wealth, he urges: "See and feel and believe yourself already in possession of the money."

You need to do the same thing when it comes to fitness. Don't just wish for it. See yourself as you want to be, not as you are. Sit quietly and close your eyes for just a few minutes a day, and imagine how you'll look and feel.

Men reading this, what do you see? A smiling, trim version of yourself strolling down the beach shirtless and confident, with big arms, powerful shoulders, and defined abs? Women: Do you see yourself pulling out of the bottom drawer of your dresser the bikini that's been hiding in there ever since you outgrew it? Have you been wishing that one day you could get it out of that drawer, put it on, and be happy and proud to let the whole world see you in it without the slightest hesitation?

BEGIN TO SEE YOUR LIFE AS YOU WANT IT TO BE

The more energy you focus on visualizing your goal, the closer you'll come to realizing it. Keeping your goal list with you will give it more power; its presence will begin to bend your thoughts and actions both consciously and unconsciously, and give your goal such momentum that it will eventually take on a life of its own. I know it may seem hard to believe, but there will come a point when it will actually be easier to carry on and see your goal through than to set it aside and cease working toward it.

Of course, physically shredding fat and adding muscle to your body require more than just visualization. There are myriad physiological factors that need to be taken into account, and we'll get there. But there's a reason I put visualization first. You can know everything there is to know about the human body, including the best way to eat and the best way to train, but if you don't believe beyond a shadow of a doubt that you can achieve your ultimate goal, then nothing else will matter. If you don't know *why* you want it—not just to look better, but to feel better about yourself and everything you do—then the goal is doomed.

Look deep inside yourself. Find the courage to acknowledge exactly where you are—then find the nerve to refuse to accept it.

LOVE THE PROCESS

Write those three words down in big letters on a sheet of paper and tape it to your fridge. It's going to go up next to your goal, because those three words are perhaps the most important three words in this book.

Thus far, we've talked a lot about goals—and with good reason. You need a point to aim at, an ideal to strive toward to get yourself moving in the right direction. But it's a grievous mistake to think of your goal as an end point or destination.

Instead, consider your goal a state of being.

Once you've lost your belly, is the work over? You shouldn't need me to tell you that it isn't. Your new lifestyle has just begun. It's commendable to achieve a high level of fitness; but to me there's nothing sadder than seeing someone reach that state, only to regress back to the beginning and have to start all over again. I've seen it happen plenty of times, and it literally pains me. I want to scream, "You were there! You had it by the short hairs! How could you let it go?!"

A good example of this phenomenon is what happens to some contestants who win *The Biggest Loser.* Here you have morbidly obese individuals who are put on a crash diet and extreme exercise regimen and undergo a dramatic transformation in a relatively short period of time. But once they get there, they often lose their grip on it, mistakenly believing they've "earned" the right to get lax with their exercise and eating habits.

I'm not wagging my finger at *The Biggest Loser.* I actually think it's a phenomenal show, and the transformations are quite inspiring—it's a shining example to people everywhere that nothing is impossible. My only question is: Within that process, what have the contestants learned about sustainability? What have they learned that they can take with them and use for the rest of their lives? Many of them make the mistake of becoming so focused on the end result that they fail to learn to love the process of getting there. The goal isn't viewed as a state of being but as an end point—and that sets the stage for regression and failure.

So, understand as you begin this journey that putting in the work in the gym and in the kitchen isn't the whole story. It's not enough to train hard and eat your vegetables if you're hating every second of it and can't stop thinking about how much you'd rather be watching a movie with a big box of Milk Duds in your lap.

You need to learn to love the feeling of the iron in your hands when you go to the gym, and imagine your muscles getting stronger as you lift the weight—not fly through the sets because you can't wait to get home and crap out on the couch.

You need to learn to love the taste of broccoli, cauliflower, kale, and spinach, and savor those tastes because the nutrients they're providing your body are going to give you long-lasting energy, prevent disease, and make you whole.

You need to accept this fact and believe it in your heart of hearts.

If you can't do that for yourself, and truly learn to love the process of becoming fit, then expect to lead a life that's riddled with disappointment and failure, and to experience success only in fits and starts.

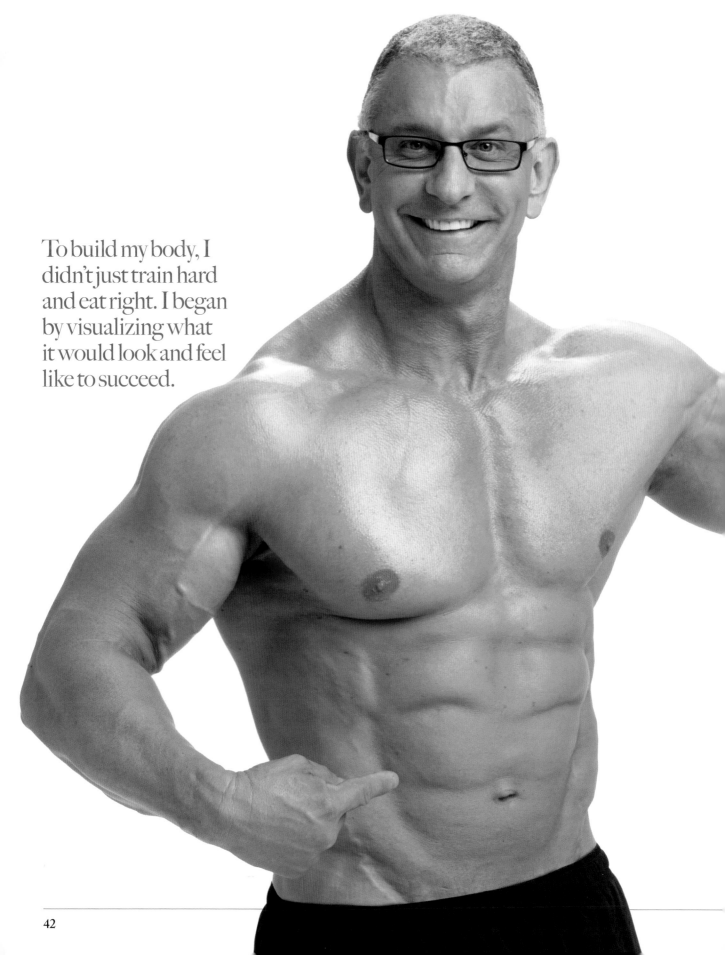

To build my body, I didn't just train hard and eat right. I began by visualizing what it would look and feel like to succeed.

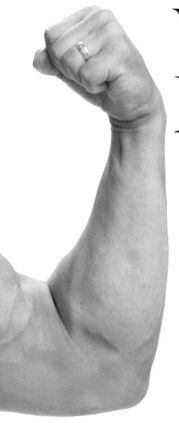

Work Your Mind Like a Muscle

Success Tactic No. 3

THE IDEA OF THE MIND-MUSCLE CONNECTION gained prevalence with the rise of bodybuilding in the 1960s and '70s. In essence, the mind-muscle connection is created when a lifter concentrates all his mental energy on the lift he's doing at that moment. For example, he doesn't just do a biceps curl—he does it and at the same time imagines what's going on inside the muscle as the weight is lifted, the blood rushing to the working muscle fibers to deliver the nutrients that will foster growth.

Arnold Schwarzenegger, for one, took this concept a step further, going through an entire workout in his mind before hitting the gym, envisioning every rep of every exercise and imagining his muscles growing in the process.

Whether you believe it's possible to mentally grow your muscles and slash your body fat with the power of your mind is irrelevant. There's inherent value in being in the present moment rather than simply going through the motions. Think of how you perform at work when you're involved in a project that truly excites you and appeals to your interests. Now think of how you perform when you just want the task to be over and done with. The difference is as stark as night and day—or, in our case, fat and fit.

In addition to being a tremendously helpful tool for keeping you focused, the mind-muscle connection is also your best weapon for combating the oppressiveness a long-term goal can begin to exert on your psyche. It's very common to start out strong on a training program, make a small amount of progress over a couple of weeks, then become overwhelmed when you think about the sustained effort it's going to take to reach your ultimate goal. The mind-muscle connection is really just another way of keeping your mind in the present.

In one of my favorite movies, *The Empire Strikes Back,* Yoda dispenses some poignant advice to Luke Skywalker. I've been in more than one gym with Yoda quotes on the walls, the most popular being: "Do. Or do not. There is no try." I love that quote, but there's one I love even more. Yoda implores his pupil, Luke, to keep his mind on the task at hand. Referring to him in the third person, he says: "All his life has he looked away, to the future, to the horizon. Never his mind on where he was! What he was doing!" Watching Yoda poke Luke in the chest while he delivers these lines is both hilarious and inspiring. Who would have thought that a little green puppet could teach us so much?

You, too, need to follow his advice: Keep your mind on where you are and what you're doing.

Success Tactic No. 4

Consider the Gym Your Friend

THE GYM HAS BEEN A REFUGE for me through the years. Whenever I come upon hard times in my life, I know I can take the negative energy that's building up inside me and bring it to the gym to turn it into something positive.

That was the case in 2008, when I (as it turned out, temporarily) lost my job at Food Network. In the month between being let go and being rehired, I spent two to three hours in the gym every single day, never taking a day off. I was frustrated and disappointed, but determined not to let a setback become a true failure. So instead of sulking and wishing for another chance, I went into the gym and attacked my workouts. A comeback, I believed, could start with my body—so I took a major negative change in my life and worked to turn it into a positive one.

I know from a life lived in the gym that this is the case for a lot of us. But too many times we go work out *only* when we're troubled. A survey taken in the U.S. during the recession that followed the 2008 housing collapse found that gym visits actually spiked dramatically around this time. I interpret this to mean that once people lost their jobs, they, like me, decided to take more time for themselves, to try and get their health back on track. And while it's encouraging to hear a statistic like that, it's also troubling: Why should it take the loss of a job to finally get us to the gym? Why shouldn't the gym also be a place to go when we're feeling happy and satisfied with life, and have a steady income?

Instead of going to the gym only when we've got frustrations to vent, why not go when we've got good vibes to share?

Everyone's busy. None of us is ever going to "find" the time. If it's a priority, we *make* the time. I understand that for most people, their families and their jobs are their top priorities in life. But if you love your family—and want to be at your best at work—then make time for the gym. Great relationships and top job performance depend on keeping yourself healthy.

Hard training and a clean diet truly are the starting points for success in all areas of your life.

+ IRON REFUGE

In good times and bad, the gym is always there for you—unchanging, offering a standing invitation to you to come in and better yourself.

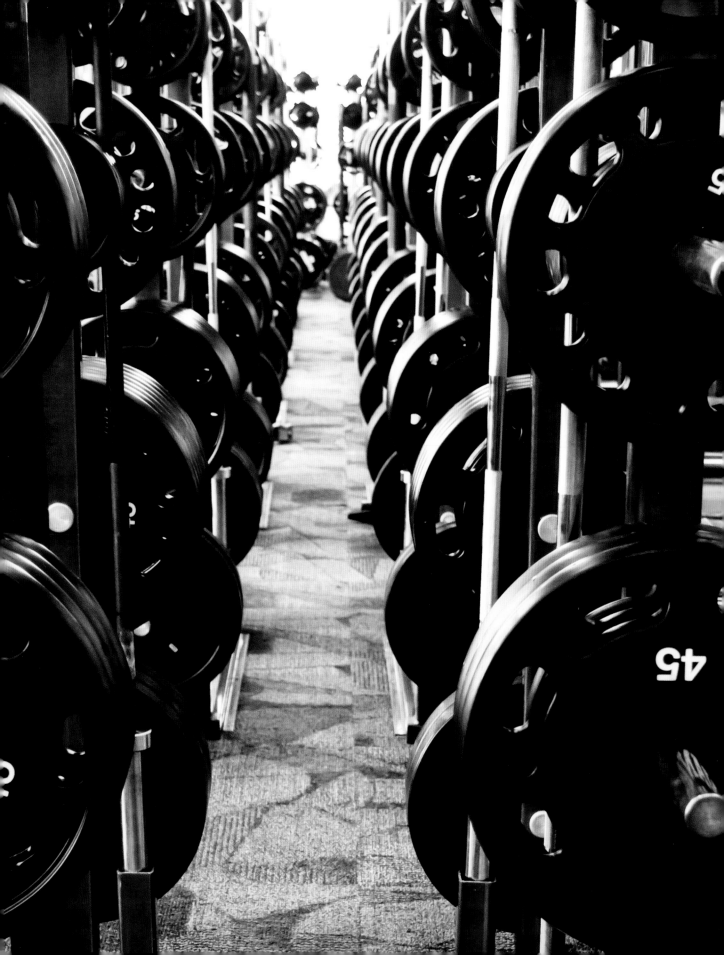

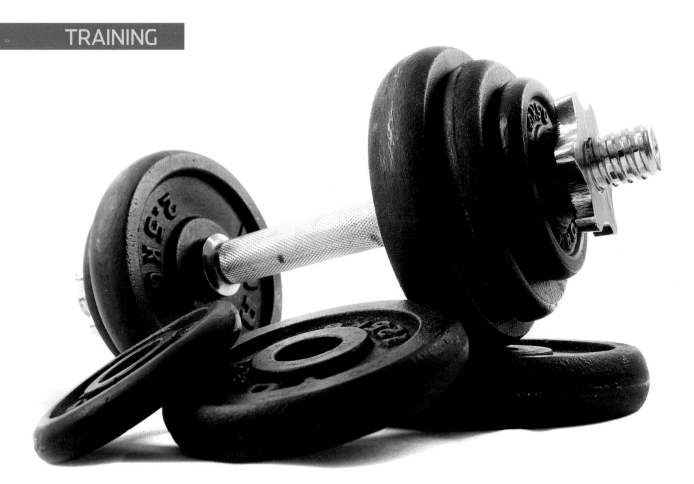

Success Tactic No. 5

Don't Get Fancy— Just Stick with the Basics

THE TRAINING PROGRAM PRESENTED on the following pages is the very same workout I used during my first 20-plus years in the gym. It's a simple body-part split that, when done at high intensity with minimal rest between sets, will allow you to build muscle. Increasing muscle mass will, over time, increase your metabolism. And the short rest periods—about 90 seconds between sets—will help burn fat.

If you're a beginner, all the instructions you need are here. If you're not, this might look familiar—that said, don't discount it. You don't need something new and exotic to get yourself in great shape. No special equipment or branded training programs—just the fundamentals, combined with healthy eating, and nothing more. The exercises that worked in the 1950s and '60s are the same ones that work today. No matter how every infomercial screams otherwise, the basics are all you need.

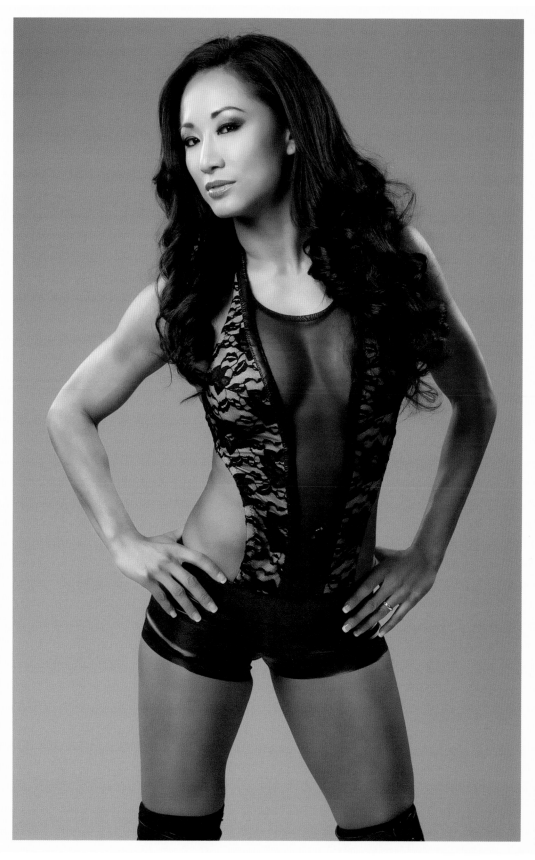

Ladies, You're Not Going to Get Big

Women have been told they need to stay away from a guy's way of training because they'll "get big" or "look like a man."

Basic biology shows this is impossible. Men and women produce different hormones that shape their bodies in distinctly different ways. In fact, it's precisely *because* of these hormonal differences that women don't need to train differently from men.

Case in point: My wife, Gail, uses the same exercises I do. Have a look at the picture to the left. Is she manly? I certainly wouldn't say so. She's lean and athletic. There's no amount of lifting that could ever make her look like a man. I beg you to hear this point: You will not get too big. It's just not going to happen. The female bodybuilders you're worried you'll end up resembling have been at it for years, eating huge amounts of food—and sometimes taking a lot of anabolic drugs—to cause those sorts of changes in their bodies.

Men and women have the same structural needs. We need strength in all areas of our bodies, so it behooves us to choose the most effective exercises to build that strength. These are the exercises you'll see in my training program. They are not gender-specific.

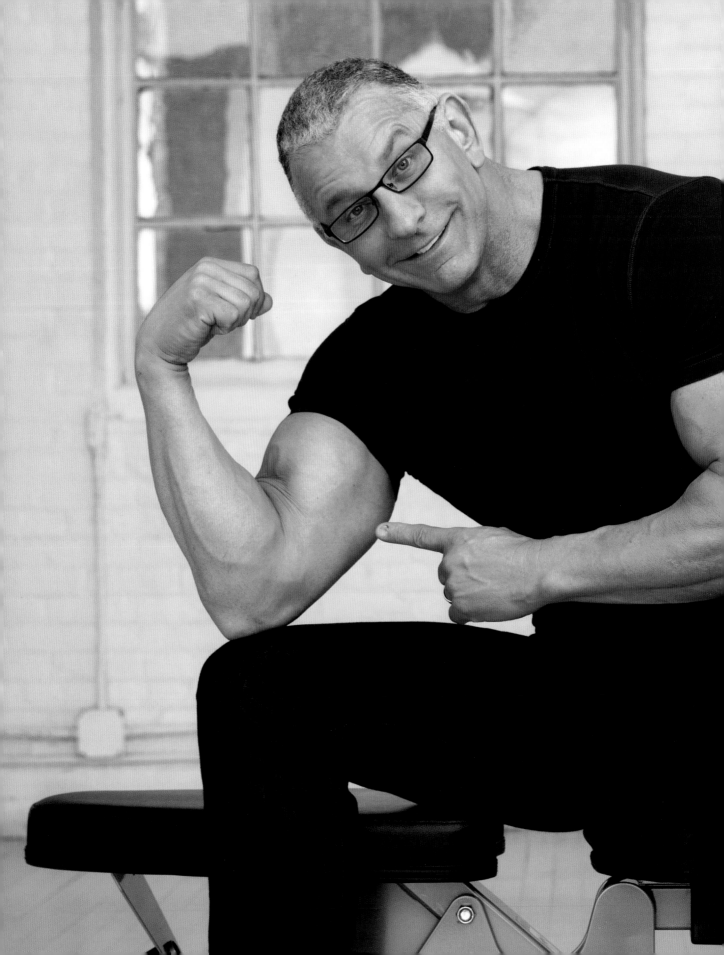

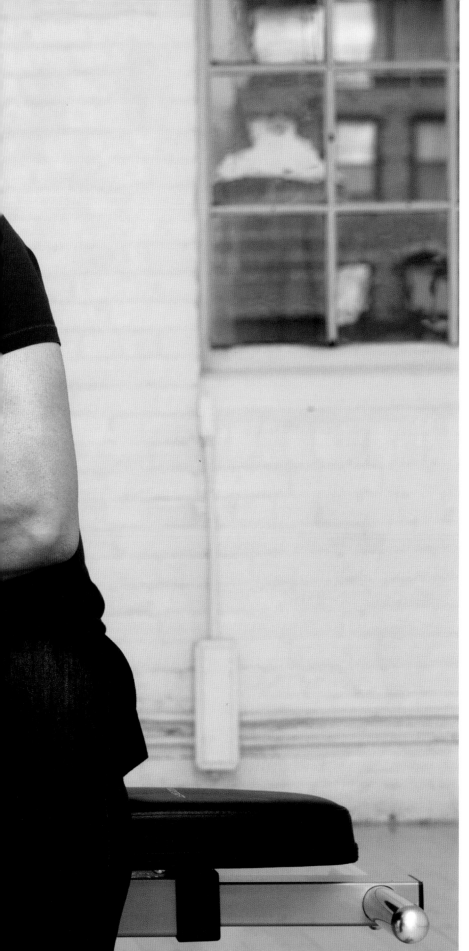

It may seem like sheer vanity, but liking the way you look will have a tremendously positive carryover effect on the rest of your life.

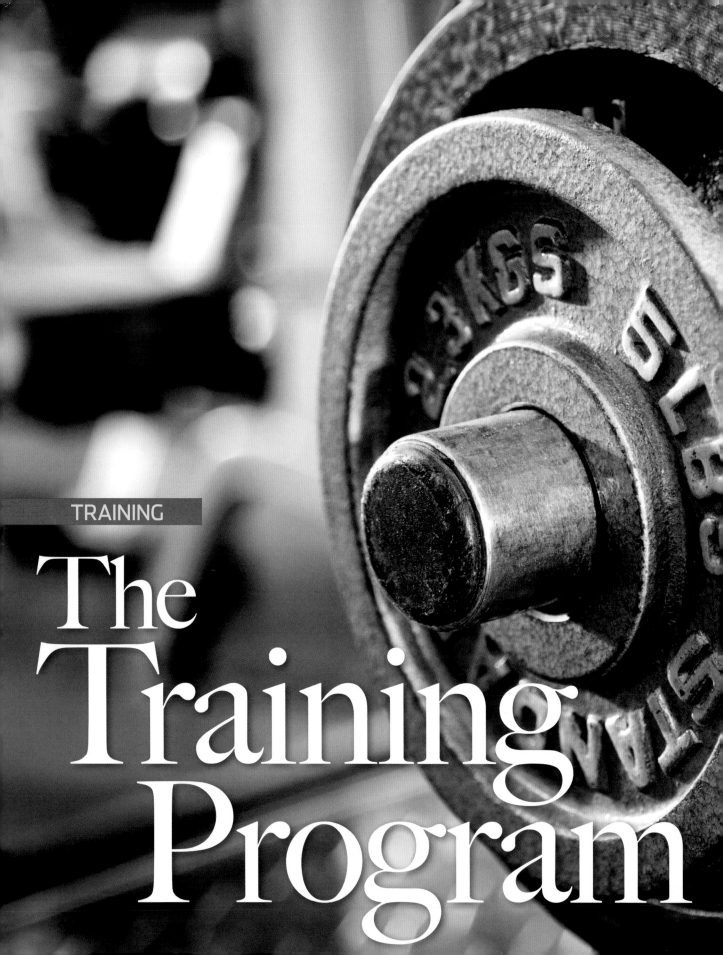

The Training Program

Weekly Workout Split

Directions: Perform each workout once a week. Your actual schedule may vary, so the days of the week I've listed here are just suggestions. Abs are done three times a week; you can find the abs routine on page 74. This is the same basic body-part split I've followed for more than 20 years, so I'm walking proof that it can be followed in perpetuity with excellent results. It's completely scalable, too, so don't feel any pressure to use the kind of weights I'm using in the photos. Pick weights that challenge you, but that you can still move safely. And if this looks too intimidating, find my Starter's Program on page 76.

Monday	I	Chest, Cardio, Abs
Tuesday	II	Back, Cardio
Wednesday	III	Legs, Abs
Thursday		Off
Friday	IV	Shoulders, Cardio
Saturday	V	Arms, Cardio, Abs
Sunday		Off/Light Cardio

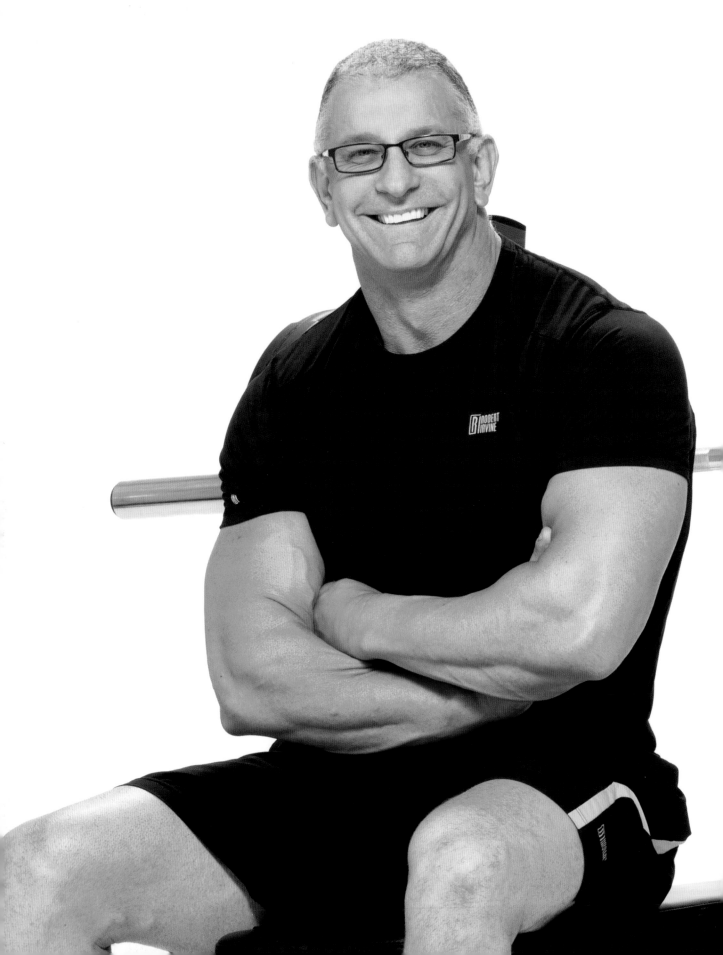

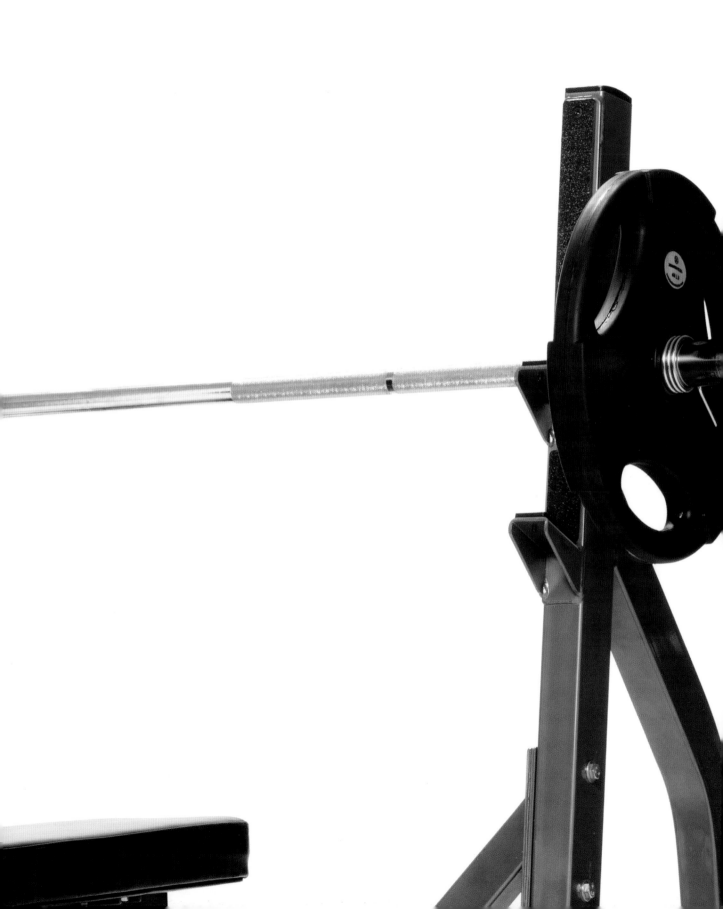

Chest

Cardio: Perform 20 minutes of cardio on an elliptical or other machine of your choice. Get your heart rate up between 70% and 80% of your maximum heart rate, or MHR. (SEE THE MHR CALCULATOR ON PG. 89.)

Targeted Warmup
Arm Circle, 2 x 25

Grab a pair of 2½- or 5-pound plates and extend your arms straight out to your sides, spinning your arms in small circles for 25 controlled reps. Rest, then do 25 large circles.

EXERCISE	SETS	REPS
Barbell Bench Press	4	10–12
Incline Dumbbell Press	4	12–15
Pec Flye	4	12–15
Pushup on Barbell	4	12–15
Dumbbell Pullover	4	12–15
Abs Circuit	See page 74	

Rest about 90 seconds between sets.

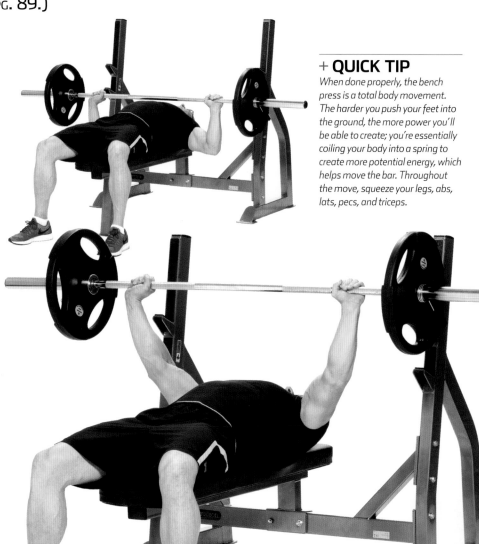

+ QUICK TIP
When done properly, the bench press is a total body movement. The harder you push your feet into the ground, the more power you'll be able to create; you're essentially coiling your body into a spring to create more potential energy, which helps move the bar. Throughout the move, squeeze your legs, abs, lats, pecs, and triceps.

▶ Barbell Bench Press
4 Sets x 10–12 Reps

Lie on a bench with your feet flat on the floor. Squeeze your shoulder blades together, and grasp the bar with a slightly wider than shoulder-width grip, wrapping your thumbs securely around the bar. With the help of a spotter, unrack the bar and lower it under control, contracting your lats throughout the movement. Pushing with your lats, triceps, and pecs, drive the bar back to the starting position.

Incline Dumbbell Press *4 Sets x 12–15 Reps*

Set a bench to a 45-degree angle. Lie back with a pair of dumbbells on your knees. "Kick" each dumbbell up to shoulder level, using your knees to assist the weights into the starting position. Push the weights straight up until your elbows are locked out. Lower them slowly to return to the starting position.

Pec Flye *4 Sets x 12–15 Reps*

Lie down on a flat bench and press a pair of dumbbells straight up over your chest. Keeping your elbows fully extended, slowly spread your arms apart until they're at your sides, parallel to the floor. Contract your pecs as you bring the weights back to the starting position. Squeeze your pecs for a second before starting the next rep.

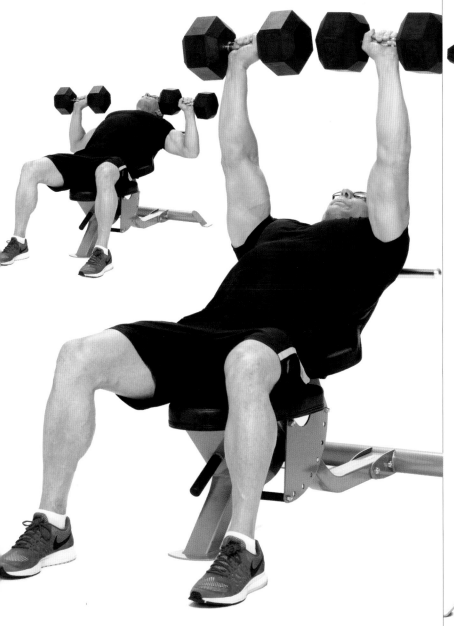

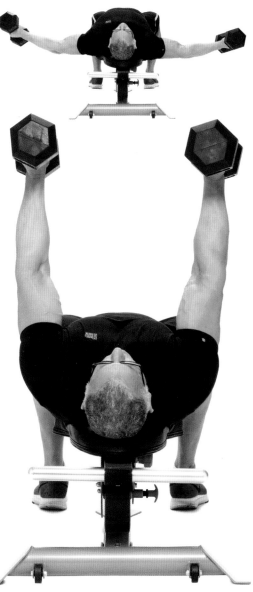

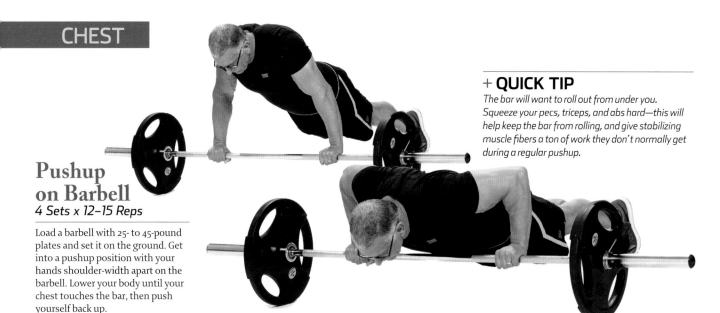

+ QUICK TIP

The bar will want to roll out from under you. Squeeze your pecs, triceps, and abs hard—this will help keep the bar from rolling, and give stabilizing muscle fibers a ton of work they don't normally get during a regular pushup.

Pushup on Barbell
4 Sets x 12–15 Reps

Load a barbell with 25- to 45-pound plates and set it on the ground. Get into a pushup position with your hands shoulder-width apart on the barbell. Lower your body until your chest touches the bar, then push yourself back up.

▼ Dumbbell Pullover *4 Sets x 12–15 Reps*

Lie down on a bench with your feet flat on the floor, holding a single heavy dumbbell overhead with both hands. Lower the weight behind your head, allowing it to stretch your pecs, and point the lowest part of your rib cage toward the sky. Contract your pecs and lats as you move the weight back to the starting position.

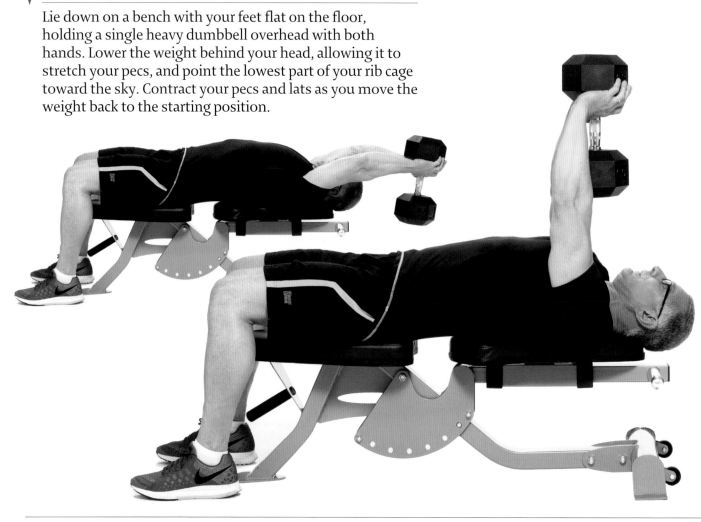

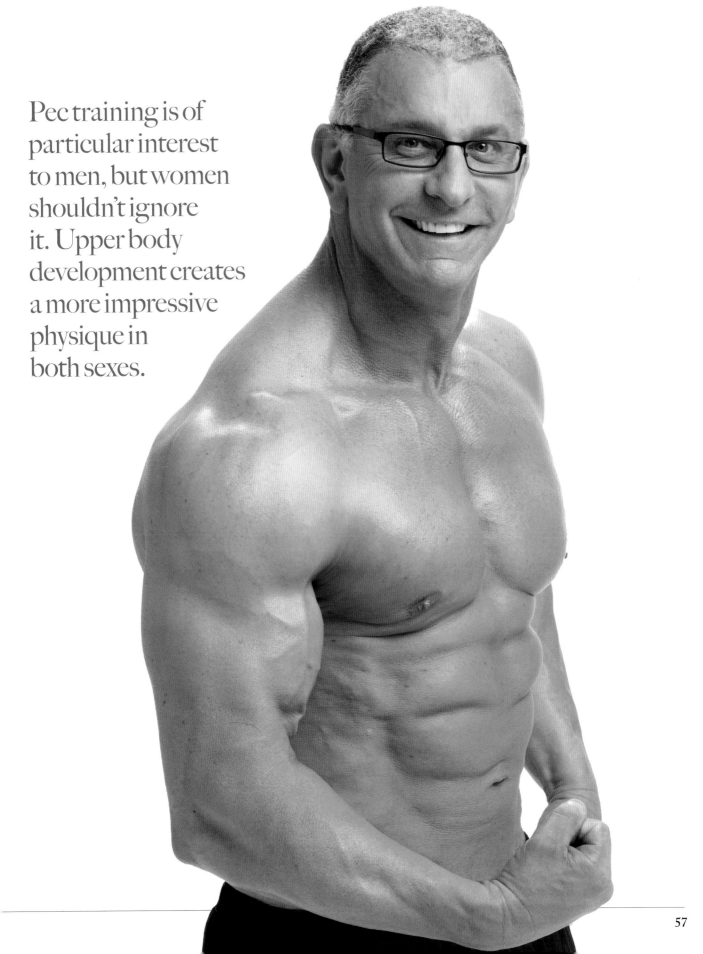

Pec training is of
particular interest
to men, but women
shouldn't ignore
it. Upper body
development creates
a more impressive
physique in
both sexes.

Back

Cardio: Perform 30 minutes of cardio on an elliptical or other machine of your choice. Get your heart rate up between 65% and 75% of your maximum heart rate, or MHR.

Targeted Warmup

Band Pull-apart, 2 x 25

Grab an elastic band with both hands and pull it apart, initiating the move from your shoulder blades. The band will stretch across your chest until both arms are fully extended. Slowly return to the start position.

Bodyweight Squat, 2 x 25

Stand with your feet slightly wider than shoulder-width apart and both hands in front of you or behind your head. Squat low to the ground, making sure your thighs get at least parallel to the floor. Engage your glutes as you stand back up.

EXERCISE	SETS	REPS
Deadlift	4	8–10
One-arm Cable Row	4	12–15 (each side)
Lat Pulldown	4	12–15
Straight-arm Pulldown	4	12–15
One-arm Dumbbell Row	4	12–15 (each side)
Bentover Barbell Row	4	10

Rest about 90 seconds between sets.

Deadlift
4 Sets x 8–10 Reps

Stand in front of a loaded barbell with your feet shoulder-width apart. Squat low to grab the bar with an alternating grip—one hand overhand, one hand underhand. Keep your back flat and eyes forward as you drive your heels into the floor to stand up.

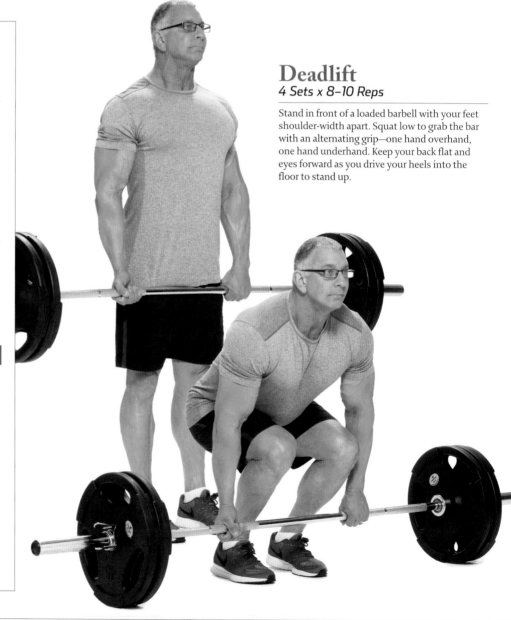

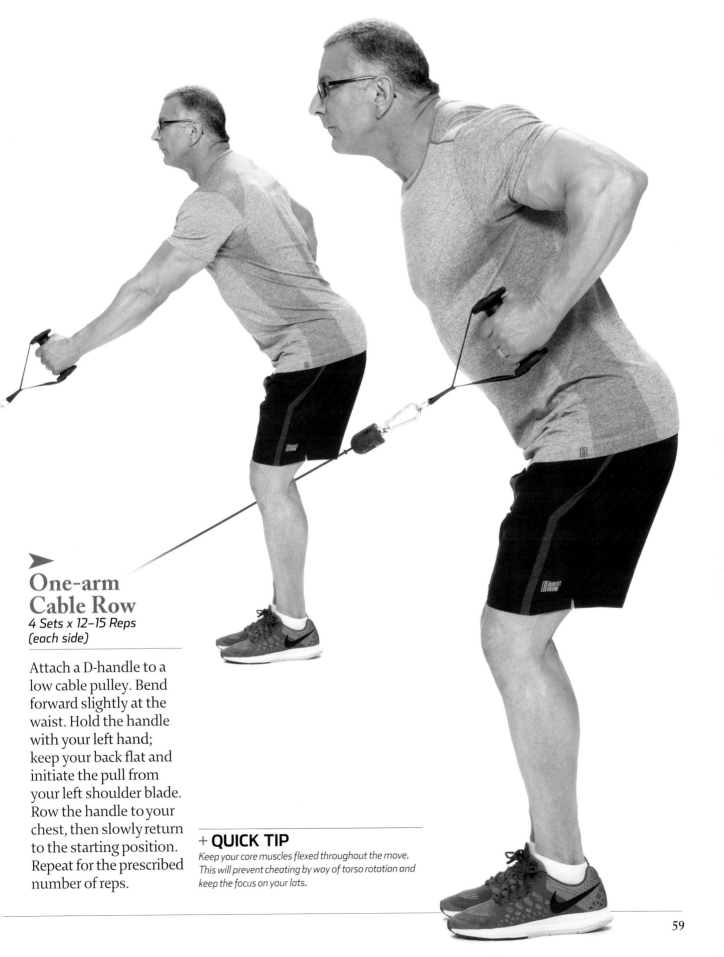

One-arm Cable Row
4 Sets x 12–15 Reps (each side)

Attach a D-handle to a low cable pulley. Bend forward slightly at the waist. Hold the handle with your left hand; keep your back flat and initiate the pull from your left shoulder blade. Row the handle to your chest, then slowly return to the starting position. Repeat for the prescribed number of reps.

+ QUICK TIP
Keep your core muscles flexed throughout the move. This will prevent cheating by way of torso rotation and keep the focus on your lats.

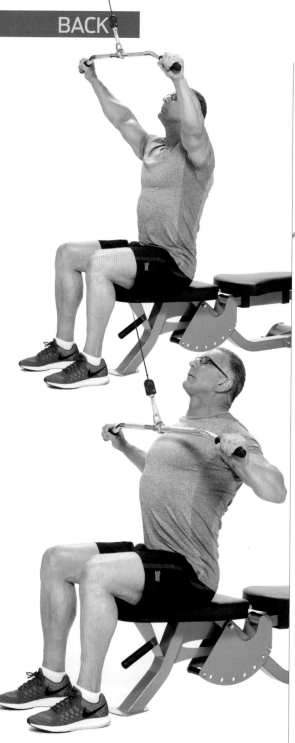

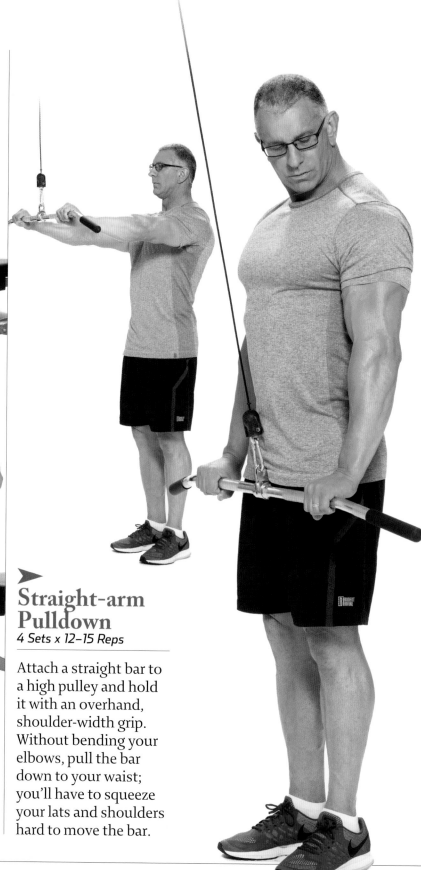

Lat Pulldown
4 Sets x 12–15 Reps

Sit facing the weight stack at a lat pulldown station. Grab the bar with a wide grip and pull it down to your chest, initiating the pull with your shoulder blades.

➤ Straight-arm Pulldown
4 Sets x 12–15 Reps

Attach a straight bar to a high pulley and hold it with an overhand, shoulder-width grip. Without bending your elbows, pull the bar down to your waist; you'll have to squeeze your lats and shoulders hard to move the bar.

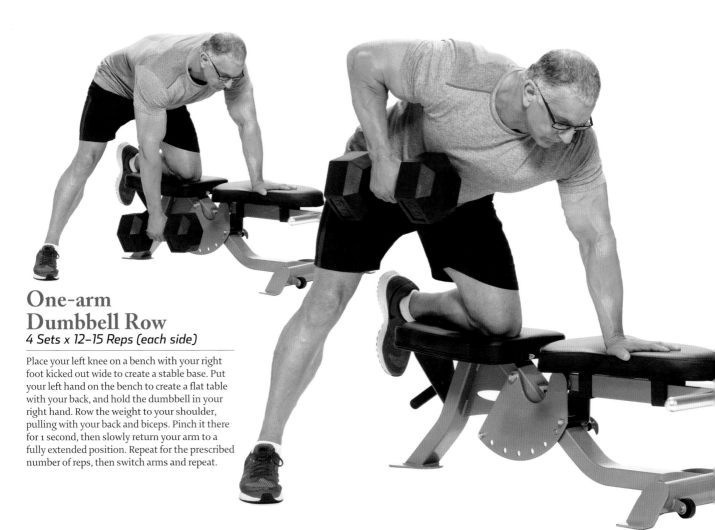

One-arm Dumbbell Row
4 Sets x 12–15 Reps (each side)

Place your left knee on a bench with your right foot kicked out wide to create a stable base. Put your left hand on the bench to create a flat table with your back, and hold the dumbbell in your right hand. Row the weight to your shoulder, pulling with your back and biceps. Pinch it there for 1 second, then slowly return your arm to a fully extended position. Repeat for the prescribed number of reps, then switch arms and repeat.

Bentover Barbell Row
4 Sets x 10 Reps

Stand holding a loaded barbell with a double overhand grip. Bend over so that your torso is leaning forward at a 45-degree angle, with the barbell hanging at your knees. Keeping your back flat, row the barbell to the base of your sternum. Hold it there for a beat, then slowly return to the starting position.

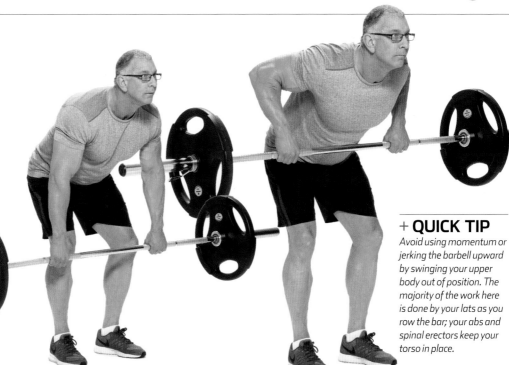

+ QUICK TIP
Avoid using momentum or jerking the barbell upward by swinging your upper body out of position. The majority of the work here is done by your lats as you row the bar; your abs and spinal erectors keep your torso in place.

Legs

General Warmup: **Perform 5–10 minutes of cardio on an elliptical or other machine of your choice.**

Targeted Warmup
Bodyweight Squat, 3 x 15

Stand with your feet slightly wider than shoulder-width apart and both hands in front of you or behind your head. Squat low to the ground, making sure your thighs get at least parallel to the floor. Engage your glutes as you stand back up.

EXERCISE	SETS	REPS
Walking Lunge	4	10 (each side)
Barbell Squat	4	8
Barbell Hip Thrust	3	12
Weighted Stepup	4	10
Quad Extension SUPERSET WITH	3	15
Prone Hamstring Curl	3	15
Standing Calf Raise	4	20
Abs Circuit	See page 74	

Rest about 90 seconds between sets.

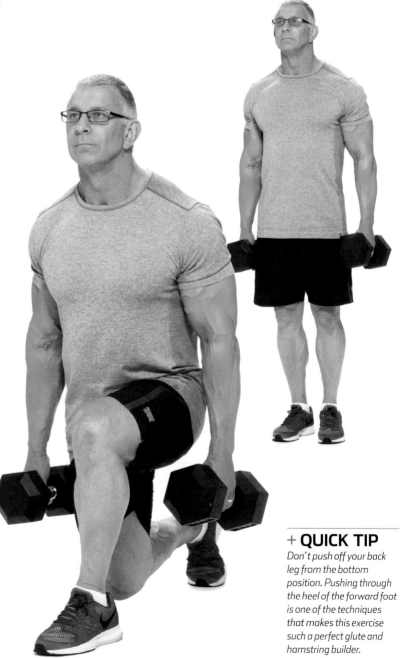

➤ Walking Lunge
4 Sets x 10 (each side)

Hold a pair of dumbbells in your hands and step forward with one foot, taking a long stride, then slowly drop your back knee to the floor. Stand back up while taking another step forward, driving through the heel of the forward foot. Keep your torso upright.

+ QUICK TIP
Don't push off your back leg from the bottom position. Pushing through the heel of the forward foot is one of the techniques that makes this exercise such a perfect glute and hamstring builder.

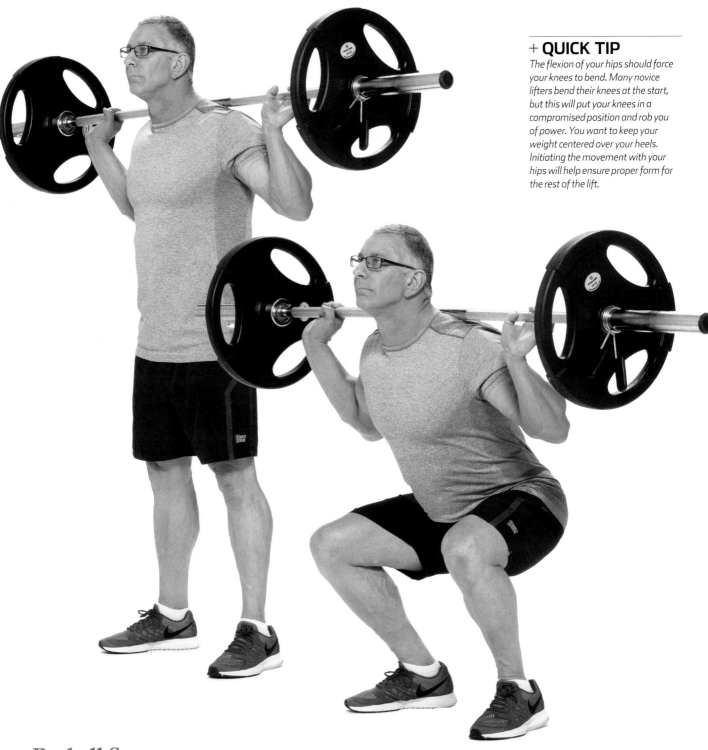

+ QUICK TIP

The flexion of your hips should force your knees to bend. Many novice lifters bend their knees at the start, but this will put your knees in a compromised position and rob you of power. You want to keep your weight centered over your heels. Initiating the movement with your hips will help ensure proper form for the rest of the lift.

Barbell Squat *4 Sets x 8 Reps*

Load a barbell in a squat rack or power rack and stand centered underneath it; the bar should cross the base of your traps at the top of your shoulder blades. Hold it in place with your hands. Keeping your head up and eyes forward, initiate the downward motion by flexing your hips—sticking your butt out in the wind. Drop your hips and bend your knees until the tops of your thighs are parallel to the floor. Keep your core muscles tight throughout the move to keep your body stable and avoid spinal injury. Flex your glutes and hamstrings as you drive your feet into the floor to stand back up.

Barbell Hip Thrust
3 Sets x 12 Reps

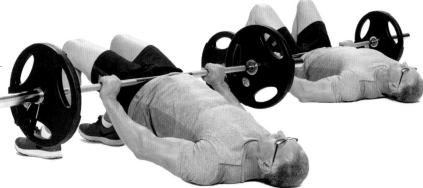

Lie on the floor faceup underneath a loaded barbell so that the center of the bar rests on your hips. (You can wrap the bar with a towel or cover your hips with cushioning, like an Airex pad.) Bend your knees so that your feet are flat on the floor. Hold the bar in place with both hands, then extend your hips to form a straight line with your torso and thighs. Squeeze your glutes and hamstrings and hold the top position for 2 seconds before slowly returning to the start.

Weighted Stepup
4 Sets x 10 Reps

Hold a pair of dumbbells and stand in front of a box or weight bench. Set one foot on the box and drive through your front heel to stand up onto the box. Step down slowly. Switch legs and repeat. That's 1 rep.

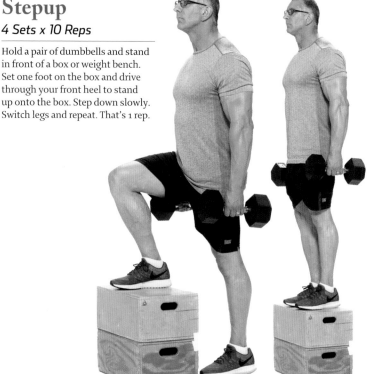

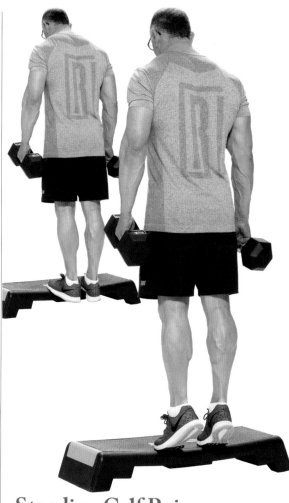

Quad Extension (not pictured) 3 Sets x 15 Reps

Adjust the footpad of a seated quad extension machine so that the pad is just at or above your ankles when you sit down. Flex your quads to extend your legs. This is a superset, so when you hit 15 reps, immediately begin hamstring curls (below).

Prone Hamstring Curl (not pictured) 3 Sets x 15 Reps

Set the footpad of a prone hamstring curl machine so that the pad is just above your ankles when you lie facedown. Contract your hamstrings to curl the weight up; get your feet as close to your butt as your range of motion will allow, and squeeze it there for 1 second. Rest 90 seconds, then go back to quad extensions.

Standing Calf Raise
4 Sets x 20 Reps

Hold a pair of dumbbells and stand with just your toes on the edge of a raised surface like a stepper or a small box. Let your heels hang down over the edge to get a good stretch in your calves. Rise onto your toes as high as you can and squeeze your calves in the peak position for at least 2 seconds. Slowly lower your heels to start the next rep.

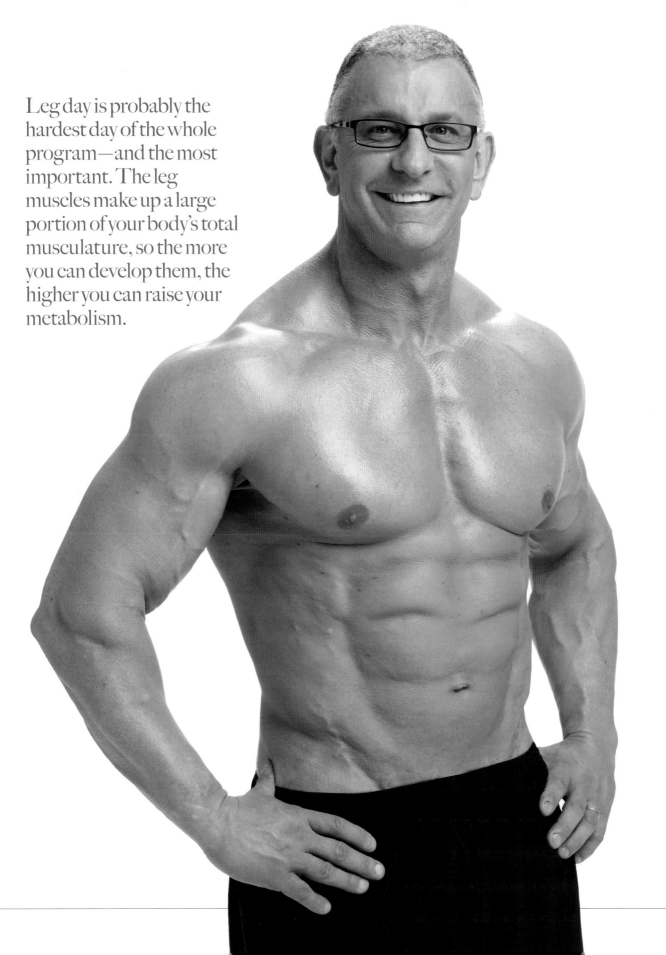

Leg day is probably the hardest day of the whole program—and the most important. The leg muscles make up a large portion of your body's total musculature, so the more you can develop them, the higher you can raise your metabolism.

Shoulders

Cardio: Perform 30 minutes of cardio on an elliptical or other machine of your choice. Get your heart rate up between 65% and 75% of your maximum heart rate, or MHR.

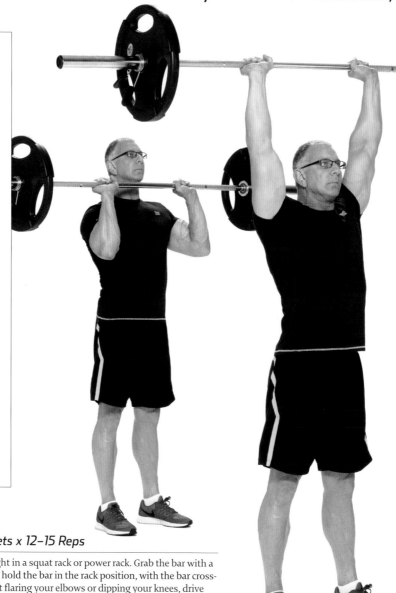

Targeted Warmup
Arm Circle, 2 x 25

Grab a pair of 2½- or 5-pound plates and extend your arms straight out to your sides, spinning your arms in small circles for 25 controlled reps. Rest, then do 25 large circles.

EXERCISE	SETS	REPS
Military Press	4	12–15
Shrug	4	12–15
GIANT SET*		
Front Raise	4	10
Lateral Raise	4	10
Upright Row	4	10
Rear Delt Flye	4	10

*Done as a continuous circuit, with no rest until after rear delt flyes.

Rest about 90 seconds between sets.

Military Press 4 Sets x 12–15 Reps

Load a barbell at about shoulder height in a squat rack or power rack. Grab the bar with a shoulder-width grip and step back to hold the bar in the rack position, with the bar crossing just above your clavicles. Without flaring your elbows or dipping your knees, drive the bar upward. Lock the bar out to full extension overhead, pushing your head forward slightly when the bar is in the topmost position. Lower the bar slowly and under control to return to the rack position.

+ QUICK TIP

Keep your core muscles flexed throughout the move. This helps prevent spinal injury and creates a strong and stable base from which to press. It also gives your abs, obliques, and spinal erectors a hefty workload. How much? A lot of strongmen have amazing six-packs, but they don't really do much direct ab work; they derive all their core strength from overhead pressing and carrying heavy objects.

Shrug *4 Sets x 12–15 Reps*

Hold a heavy barbell or a pair of heavy dumbbells and stand up straight with your core muscles flexed. Lift your shoulder girdle to pinch your shoulders up toward your ears. Flex the trapezius muscles (which extend from your neck out toward your shoulders) as you pinch at the top. Slowly lower the bar until your shoulder girdle is back in the start position.

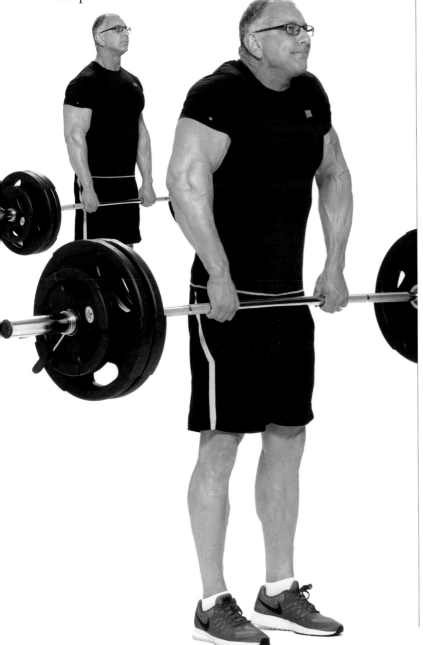

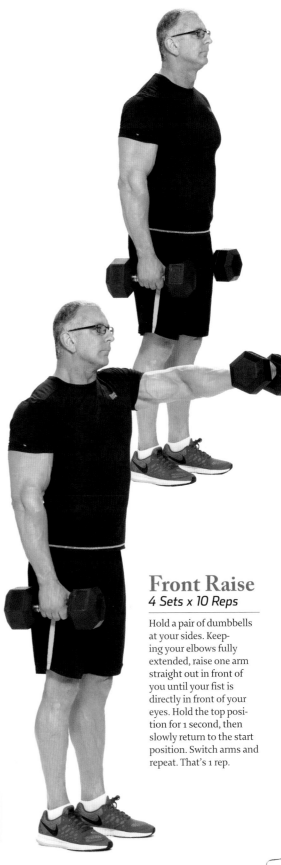

Front Raise
4 Sets x 10 Reps

Hold a pair of dumbbells at your sides. Keeping your elbows fully extended, raise one arm straight out in front of you until your fist is directly in front of your eyes. Hold the top position for 1 second, then slowly return to the start position. Switch arms and repeat. That's 1 rep.

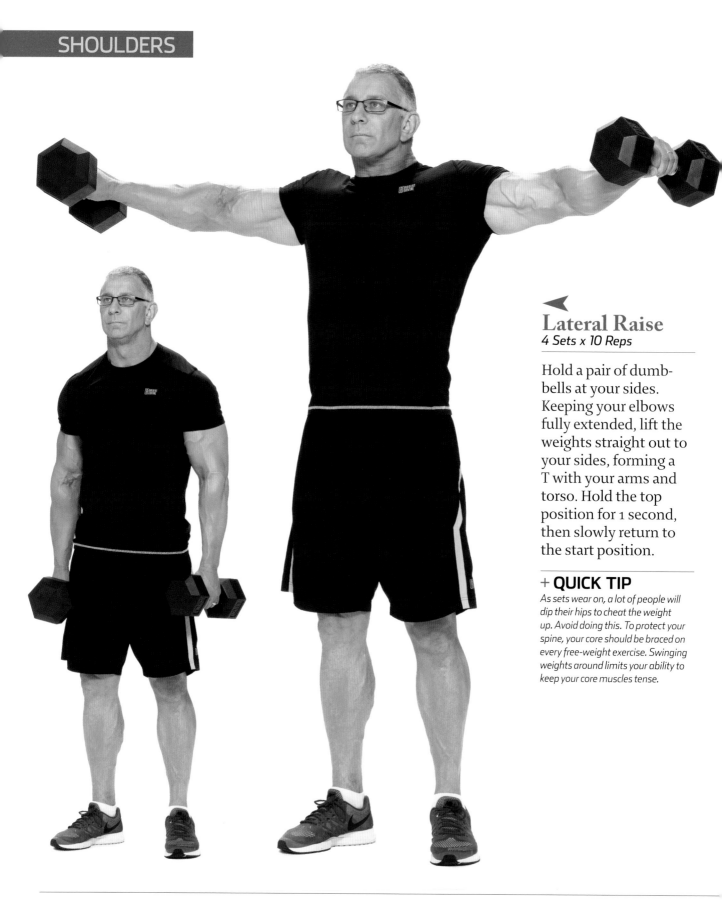

Lateral Raise
4 Sets x 10 Reps

Hold a pair of dumb-bells at your sides. Keeping your elbows fully extended, lift the weights straight out to your sides, forming a T with your arms and torso. Hold the top position for 1 second, then slowly return to the start position.

+ QUICK TIP

As sets wear on, a lot of people will dip their hips to cheat the weight up. Avoid doing this. To protect your spine, your core should be braced on every free-weight exercise. Swinging weights around limits your ability to keep your core muscles tense.

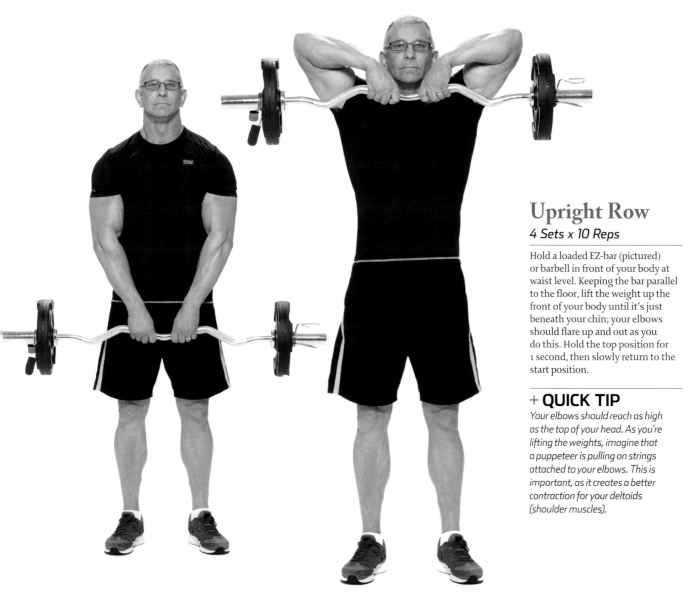

Upright Row
4 Sets x 10 Reps

Hold a loaded EZ-bar (pictured) or barbell in front of your body at waist level. Keeping the bar parallel to the floor, lift the weight up the front of your body until it's just beneath your chin; your elbows should flare up and out as you do this. Hold the top position for 1 second, then slowly return to the start position.

+ QUICK TIP

Your elbows should reach as high as the top of your head. As you're lifting the weights, imagine that a puppeteer is pulling on strings attached to your elbows. This is important, as it creates a better contraction for your deltoids (shoulder muscles).

Rear Delt Flye 4 Sets x 10 Reps

Hold a pair of dumbbells in your hands and lie facedown on an adjustable bench set to a 45-degree angle. Keeping your elbows extended, lift the dumbbells straight out to your sides to form a T with your body. Initiate the move from your shoulder blades. Hold the top position for 1 second, then slowly return to the start position.

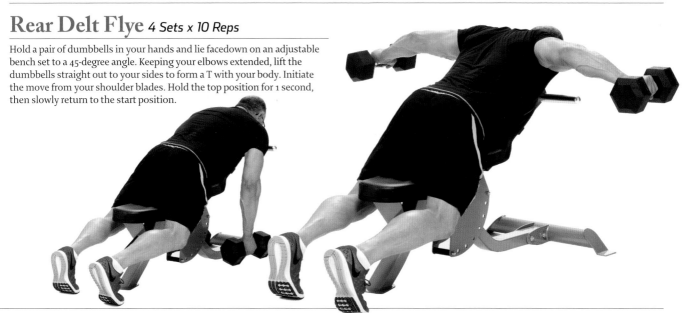

Arms

Cardio: Perform 20 minutes of cardio on an elliptical or other machine of your choice. Get your heart rate up between 70% and 80% of your maximum heart rate, or MHR.

Targeted Warmup

Barbell Curl, 5 x 50, 15, 15, 15, 50

Grab a light, fixed barbell or an empty barbell with a shoulder-width grip and curl it 50 times. Rest 1 minute, then do 15 reps with each of the following hand positions: wide, shoulder-width, and hands touching. Rest 1 more minute, then do another 50 reps at shoulder width.

EXERCISE	SETS	REPS
Hammer Curl	4	12–15
Reverse Curl	4	12–15
Cable Rope Pressdown	4	12–15
Cable Kickback SUPERSET WITH	4	12–15
Diamond Pushup	4	15
Skull Crusher SUPERSET WITH	4	12
Pushup	4	15
Abs Circuit	See page 74	

Rest about 90 seconds between sets.

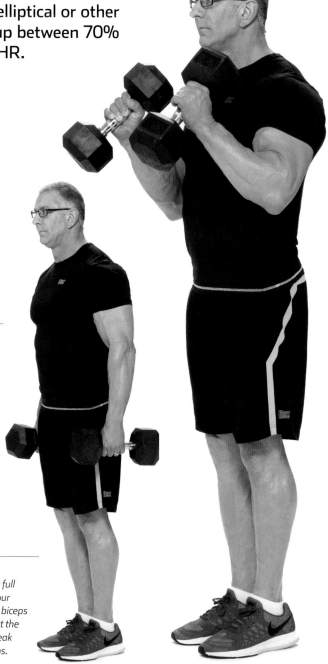

Hammer Curl

4 Sets x 12–15 Reps

Hold a dumbbell in each hand and, without using any momentum, curl the weights up to chest level, stopping just shy of your shoulders. Squeeze your biceps at the peak of the movement, then slowly return to the start position.

+ QUICK TIP

A typical hammer curl would cover a full range of motion, all the way up to your shoulders. But in that position, your biceps don't have to do any work to support the weight. Stopping just short of the peak position keeps tension on your biceps.

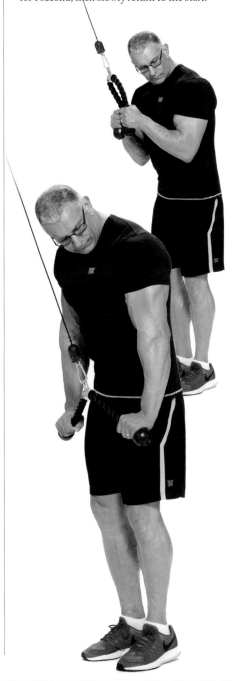

Cable Rope Pressdown
4 Sets x 12–15 Reps

Clip a rope attachment to a high pulley at a cable station and grip its ends with both hands. Keeping your elbows at your sides (imagine they're bolted to your ribs), press down, extending and contracting your triceps hard. Flare your hands out at the bottom of the movement, hold for 1 second, then slowly return to the start.

Reverse Curl
4 Sets x 12–15 Reps

Grab an EZ-bar or straight barbell with a double overhand grip and let your arms hang down to your waist. Curl the bar up using only your biceps, then slowly return to the start.

+ QUICK TIP

The awkward overhand grip is what makes this a "reverse" curl. And the special grip isn't just for show—your forearms get a lot of extra work here compared with using a traditional underhand grip.

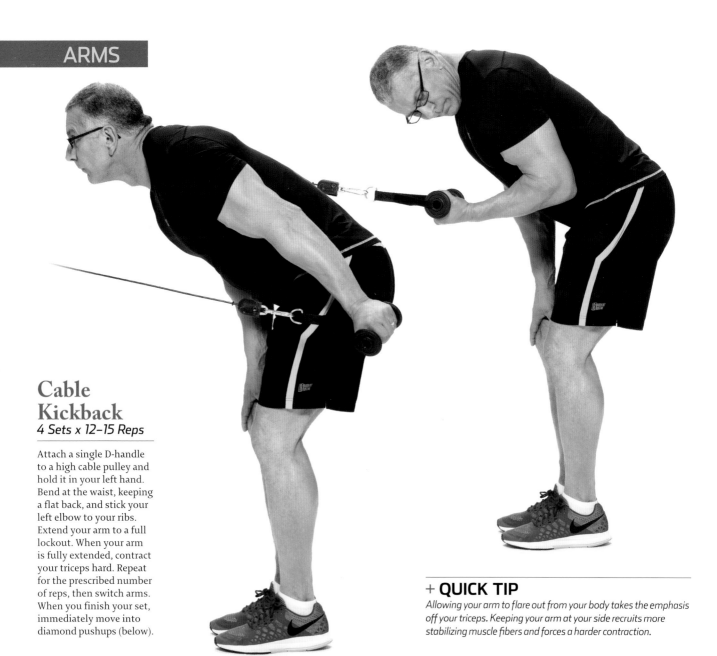

Cable Kickback
4 Sets x 12–15 Reps

Attach a single D-handle to a high cable pulley and hold it in your left hand. Bend at the waist, keeping a flat back, and stick your left elbow to your ribs. Extend your arm to a full lockout. When your arm is fully extended, contract your triceps hard. Repeat for the prescribed number of reps, then switch arms. When you finish your set, immediately move into diamond pushups (below).

+ QUICK TIP
Allowing your arm to flare out from your body takes the emphasis off your triceps. Keeping your arm at your side recruits more stabilizing muscle fibers and forces a harder contraction.

Diamond Pushup
4 Sets x 15 Reps

Get into a pushup position with your hands so close together you can touch your thumbs and index fingers to each other; the space in the middle will be in the shape of a diamond. Lower your upper body to the floor, then push up with your pecs and triceps. If a straight pushup is too difficult, modify the move by dropping to your knees. In either variation, keep your back flat. Rest about 90 seconds, then return to cable kickbacks.

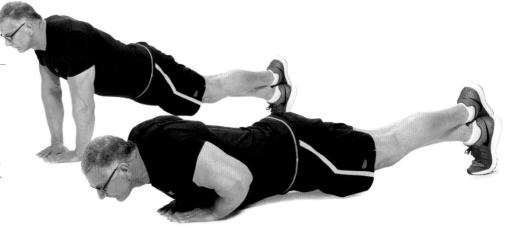

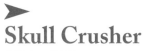

Skull Crusher
4 Sets x 12 Reps

Load an EZ-bar and lie on a flat bench with the bar in your hands. Press straight up to extend your elbows; this is the starting position. Bend your elbows to lower the bar to the top of your head. Contract your triceps hard to extend your arms. When your set is done, immediately move into pushups (below).

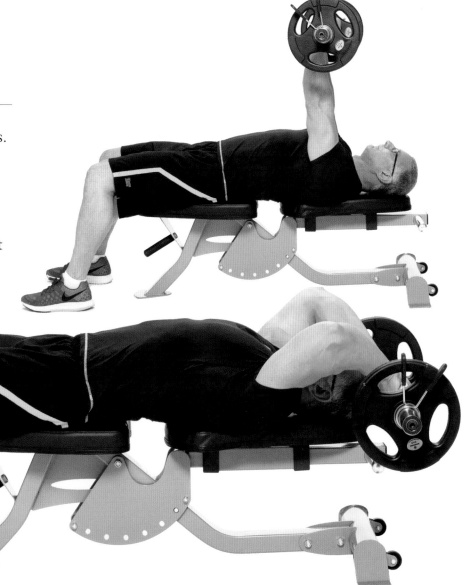

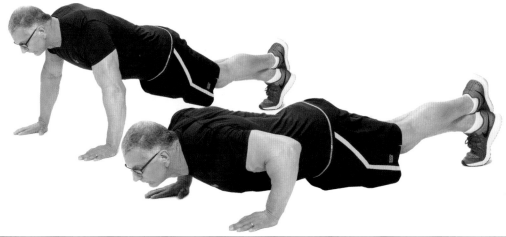

Pushup
4 Sets x 15 Reps

Get into a pushup position with your hands shoulder-width apart on the floor. Keep your back flat as you lower your body to the floor, then push back up to the start. To modify the move to add difficulty, cross your feet at the ankles, supporting your body with your hands and one foot (pictured).

Abs

Directions

Do the following ab circuit 3–4 times per week. On page 51 I recommend specific days to do this, but since there's no equipment required, you can do this at home whenever it's convenient. Perform the circuit 2–3 times through; you can start with 2 times through, then add another round after a few weeks. Another easy way to progress this workout is to add time to the planks, working up to a minute or more on the side planks and 2 minutes or more on the straight plank.

EXERCISE	REPS
Crunch	10
Bicycle Crunch	20
Leg Raise	10
Side Plank	30 sec. (each side)
Plank	60 sec.

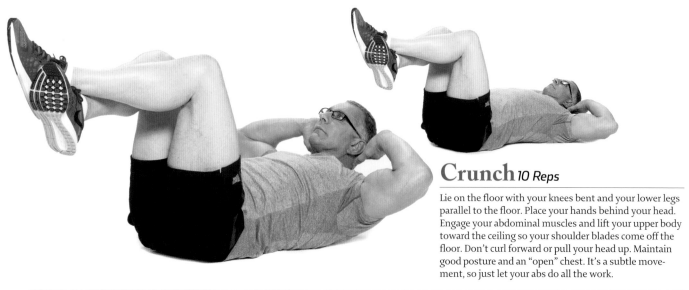

Crunch 10 Reps

Lie on the floor with your knees bent and your lower legs parallel to the floor. Place your hands behind your head. Engage your abdominal muscles and lift your upper body toward the ceiling so your shoulder blades come off the floor. Don't curl forward or pull your head up. Maintain good posture and an "open" chest. It's a subtle movement, so just let your abs do all the work.

Bicycle Crunch 20 Reps

Lie on the floor with your hands behind your head, your feet in the air, your thighs perpendicular to the floor, and your lower legs parallel to the floor. Bring one elbow across your body to meet the opposite knee; as you draw your knee toward your chest, the other leg should fully extend. That's one rep. Quickly switch sides in a cycling motion.

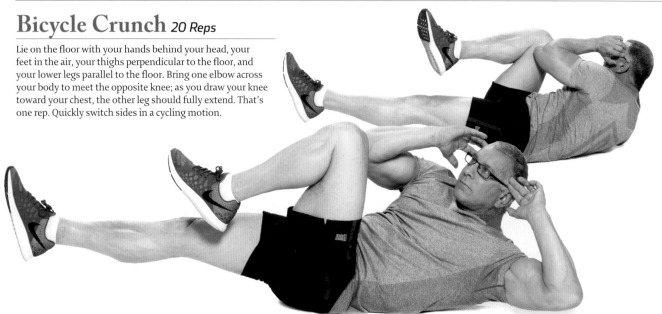

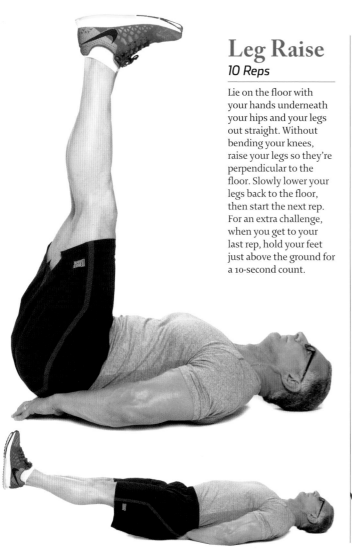

Leg Raise
10 Reps

Lie on the floor with your hands underneath your hips and your legs out straight. Without bending your knees, raise your legs so they're perpendicular to the floor. Slowly lower your legs back to the floor, then start the next rep. For an extra challenge, when you get to your last rep, hold your feet just above the ground for a 10-second count.

Side Plank 30 Seconds (each side)

Lie on your left side with your legs stacked. Lift your hips off the ground and prop yourself up on your left elbow so your body forms a straight line. Hold this position for 30 seconds, then switch sides and repeat. While you're holding the plank, squeeze the oblique muscle closest to the floor.

+ QUICK TIP

In addition to adding time, a side plank can be modified by lifting your top hand and top leg into the air. This will create an "X" frame with your body and make the move much more difficult.

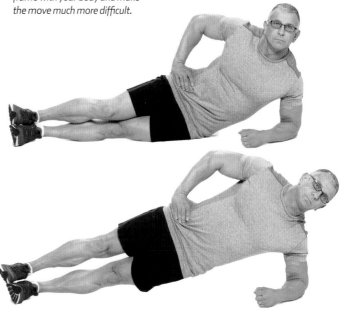

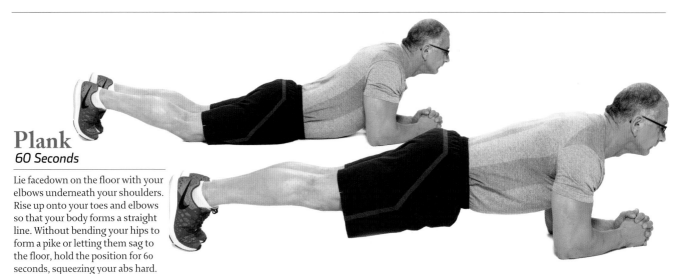

Plank
60 Seconds

Lie facedown on the floor with your elbows underneath your shoulders. Rise up onto your toes and elbows so that your body forms a straight line. Without bending your hips to form a pike or letting them sag to the floor, hold the position for 60 seconds, squeezing your abs hard.

Starter's Program

> THE FOLLOWING STARTER'S PROGRAM is intended for anyone who finds the main training program too daunting to follow right off the bat. If you're obese, suffer from high blood pressure, or have a limited range of motion that keeps you from executing some of the basic moves in the main training program, this starter's program will serve as a primer to get you mobile and fit enough to tackle the task ahead.

For the first four weeks, anything you can do, you should do. If this means just going outside and walking around your house for a few laps in the morning and a few more in the afternoon, then so be it. Whatever you can do to get blood circulating, do it! Whenever you can, stand instead of sit. Take the stairs instead of the elevator. You've probably heard this advice before, but it's solid. Moving consistently is the first part of the battle. You're in a stage right now where an hour in the gym every day can't solve all your problems. You've got to start with the little things. They're not exciting, but they add up.

As for resistance training, I want you to start doing as many bodyweight exercises as possible; I've also listed some modifications (see page 85) to help get you on your way.

The first half of each circuit is organized so it alternates upper-body and lower-body training to force the heart to supply blood to working muscles all over the body. Though it's moderate in pace, it will help you increase your heart rate so you get some cardio conditioning in while

you also strengthen your muscles.

The second half of each circuit gives you what's called "active rest" by training small muscle groups—biceps, triceps, shoulders—so you can catch your breath while still getting some work done.

Some of the moves in this starter's workout require bands. I like bands because they provide variable resistance, convenience, and portability. If you don't have any, a wide selection of great bands can be found at *performbetter.com*. Alternatively, all band moves can be replaced with light dumbbells, or with cables in a real gym.

Each circuit finishes with a plank—an abs and core exercise you'll find on page 80.

In Week 1, Circuit I should be performed 3–4 times, with a day of rest between each circuit. In Week 2, begin alternating the circuits (Monday, Circuit I; Wednesday, Circuit II; Friday, Circuit I, etc.) and continue in that fashion, eventually working up to 5 training days per week.

Total Body Circuit I

Perform all exercises without rest between them, then rest 2–4 minutes at the end of the circuit; do 2–3 total circuits.

EXERCISE	REPS
Bodyweight Squat	10
Pushup (Pg. 73)	10
Weighted Stepup (Pg. 64)	10
Band Row	10
Alternating Band Press	12
Band Pull-apart	12
French Curl	12
Plank	To Failure

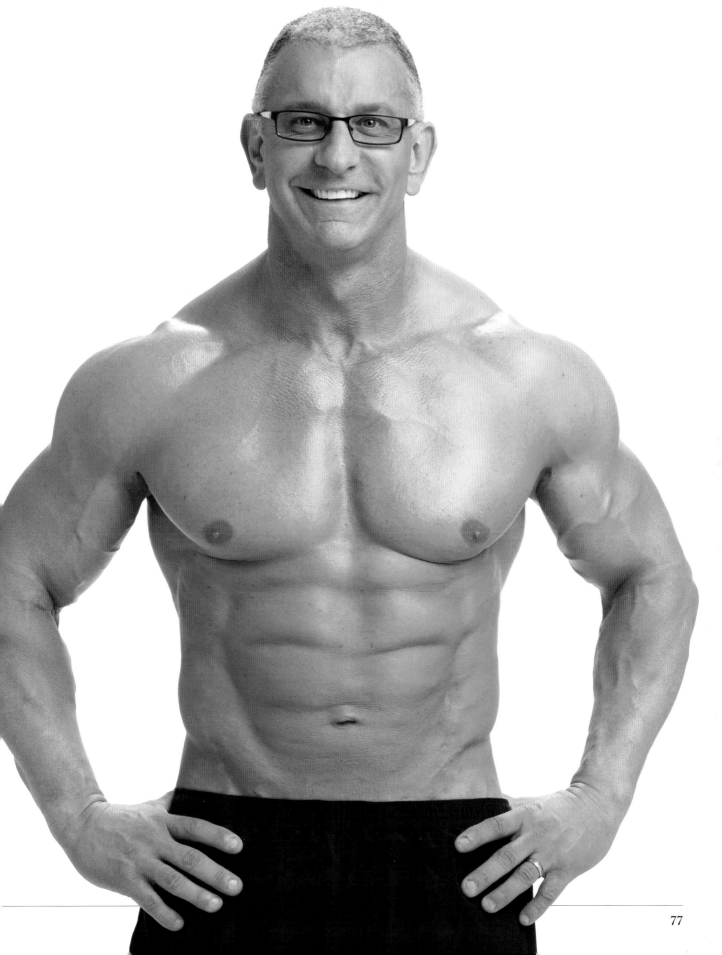

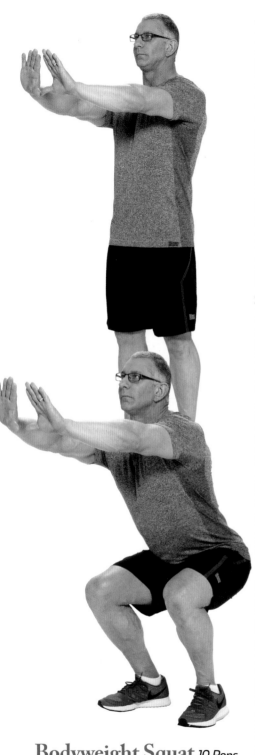

Band Row *10 Reps*

Loop a resistance band around a sturdy anchor point and hold on to both handles. Step back from the anchor point to create tension in the bands. Row the handles to your chest, squeezing your shoulder blades together for 1 second and contracting your lats. Slowly return to the start.

Bodyweight Squat *10 Reps*

With your hands straight out in front of you or resting on your hips, squat as low as you can, then stand back up.

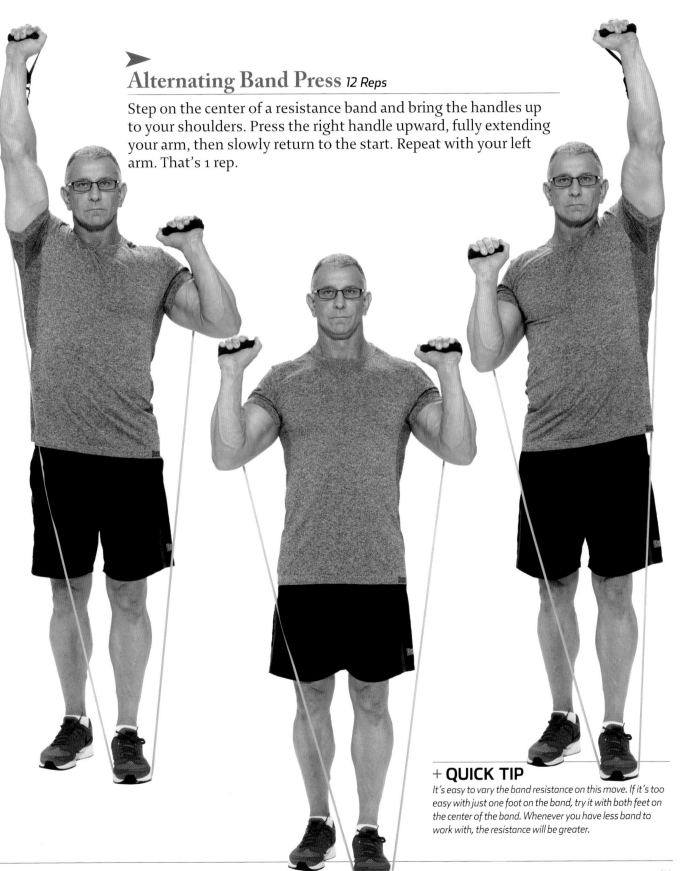

Alternating Band Press *12 Reps*

Step on the center of a resistance band and bring the handles up to your shoulders. Press the right handle upward, fully extending your arm, then slowly return to the start. Repeat with your left arm. That's 1 rep.

+ QUICK TIP

It's easy to vary the band resistance on this move. If it's too easy with just one foot on the band, try it with both feet on the center of the band. Whenever you have less band to work with, the resistance will be greater.

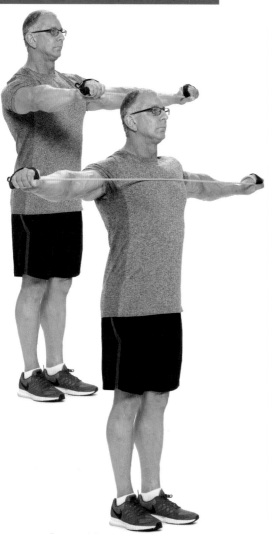

French Curl
12 Reps

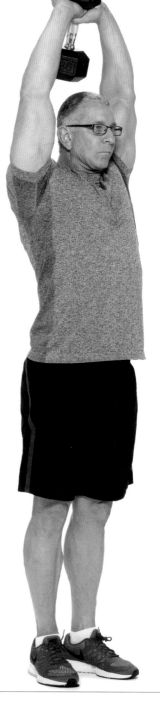

Stand or sit holding a single dumbbell overhead with both hands; the weight should be perpendicular to the floor so that your palms touch the inside of the top plate as you hold it overhead. Slowly lower the weight behind your head. Flex your triceps hard to extend your arms and press the weight overhead.

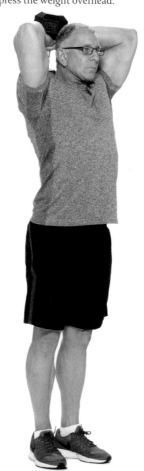

Band Pull-apart *12 Reps*

Hold on to the ends of a resistance band with your arms straight out in front of you. To create the proper tension, you can place your hands closer together, or wrap the ends of the band around your hands (pictured). With your elbows locked out, spread your arms, squeezing your shoulder blades together in the finish position. Slowly return to the start.

Plank *To Failure*

Lie facedown on the floor, propping yourself up on your toes and elbows. Keep your core muscles tight to keep your body stable and in a straight line. Hold as long as you can.

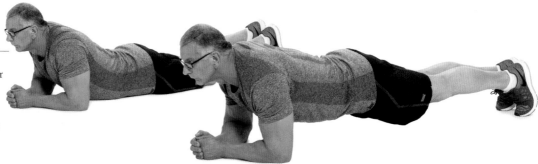

Total Body Circuit II

Perform all exercises without rest between them, then rest 2–3 minutes at the end of the circuit; do 3–4 total circuits.

EXERCISE	REPS
Wall Sit	30 seconds
Alternating Dumbbell Curl	10
Alternating Lunge	20
Dumbbell Kickback	10 (each side)
Lateral Lunge	10
Dumbbell Upright Row	15
Single-arm Chest Press	15 (each side)
Plank	To Failure

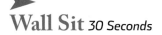

Wall Sit *30 Seconds*

Lean your upper body against a wall and drop into a sitting position, bending your knees as close to 90 degrees as possible. Hold the position for 30 seconds.

+ QUICK TIP

As you gain confidence, start pushing yourself past the 30-second mark. Once 30 seconds is manageable, increase the time by 5–10 seconds in each workout until you hit 1 minute.

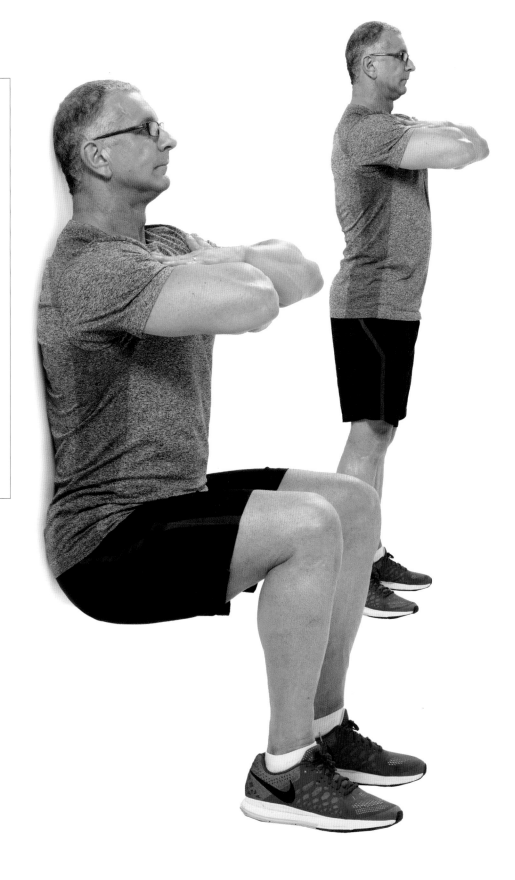

Alternating Dumbbell Curl
10 Reps

Hold a pair of dumbbells at your waist with your palms facing out. Curl a weight up to your chest, squeezing your biceps in the peak position, then lower and switch arms. That's 1 rep.

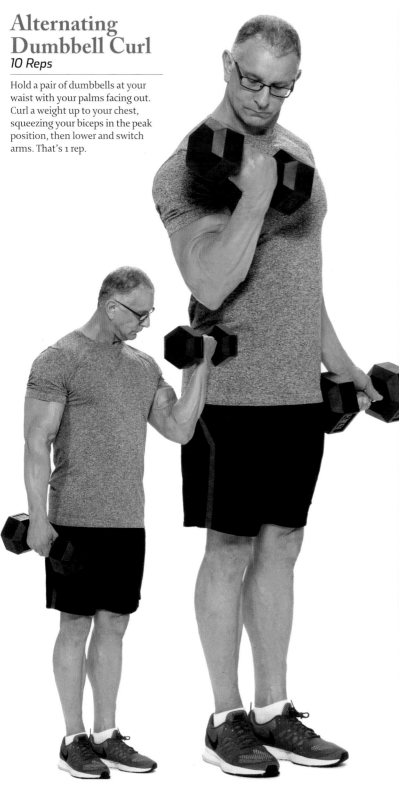

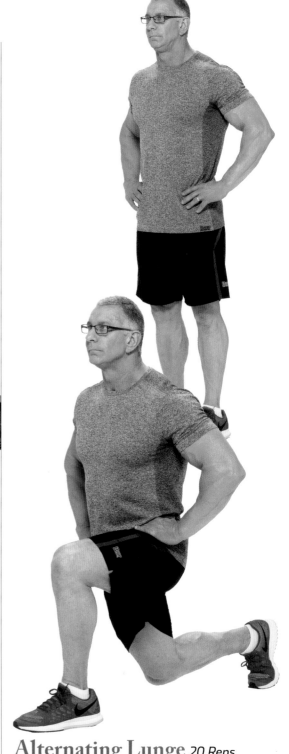

Alternating Lunge *20 Reps*

Stand with your hands on your hips and take one long stride forward with your left foot, dropping your back knee to the floor. Drive through your left heel to push yourself back up to the starting position. Alternate legs on each step.

Dumbbell Kickback

10 Reps (each side)

Place your left knee and hand on a bench to brace yourself. Hold a dumbbell in your right hand; keep your back flat. Imagine your right elbow is bolted to your hip as you reach the weight back behind you. At the finish, your arm should be parallel to the floor, elbow fully extended. Repeat for reps, then switch arms.

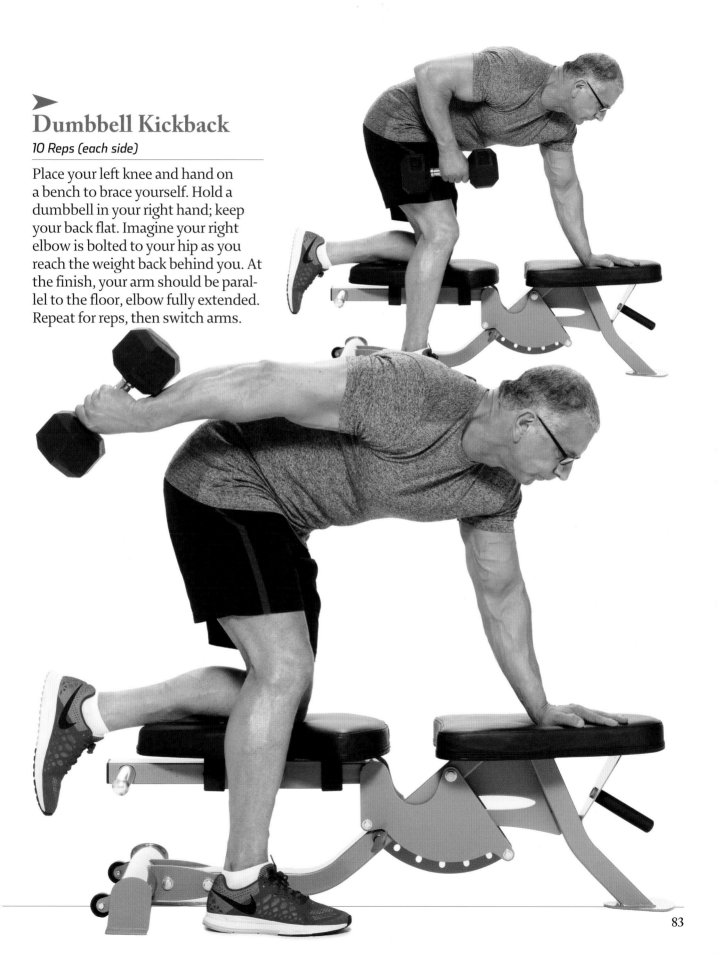

Lateral Lunge

10 Reps

Stand up straight and take a long lateral step to the left. Bend your left knee and crouch down, sinking your hips. Your right leg should be fully extended. Push through your left heel to return to the starting position, then repeat with your right leg. That's 1 rep.

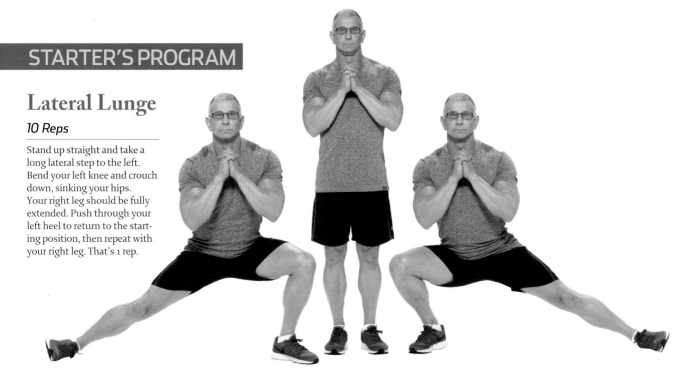

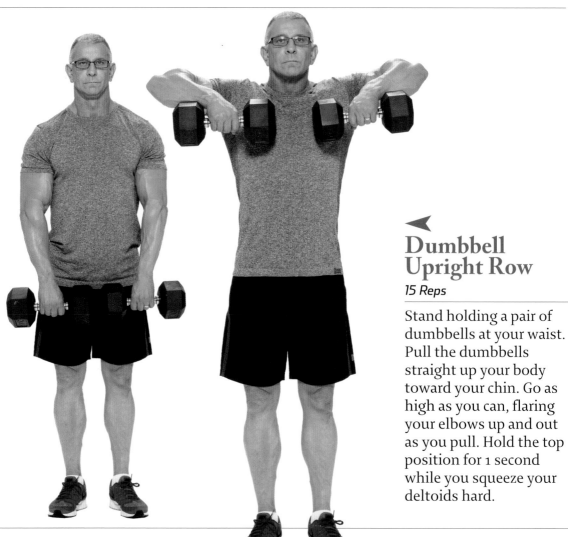

Dumbbell Upright Row

15 Reps

Stand holding a pair of dumbbells at your waist. Pull the dumbbells straight up your body toward your chin. Go as high as you can, flaring your elbows up and out as you pull. Hold the top position for 1 second while you squeeze your deltoids hard.

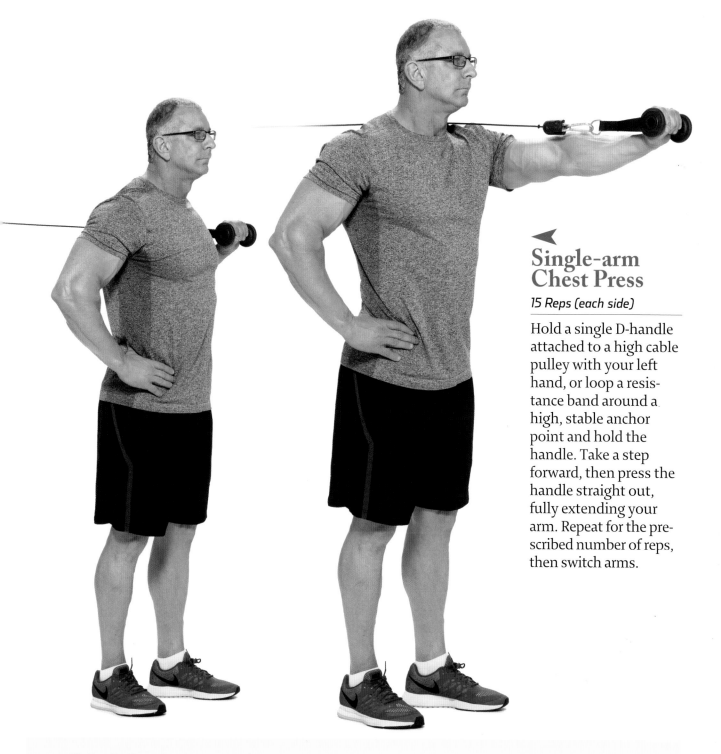

Single-arm Chest Press

15 Reps (each side)

Hold a single D-handle attached to a high cable pulley with your left hand, or loop a resistance band around a high, stable anchor point and hold the handle. Take a step forward, then press the handle straight out, fully extending your arm. Repeat for the prescribed number of reps, then switch arms.

Modifications

If you found any of the bodyweight moves in the starter's program too difficult to complete with good form, try the following modifications. Use these modified versions to build up the strength to do the regular versions shown and described in the previous pages.

➤ **Bodyweight Squat**
If you can't squat low, squat down onto a high box or bench, or into a chair. You want to build up stability and also learn the proper depth. Starting with a high box or chair and then squatting progressively lower will help tremendously. Remember: The goal as you rise out of the hole (the bottom of a squat) is to do so without any momentum. Every time you sit down, practice standing up without using your hands.

➤ **Pushup**
The progression from easiest to hardest is: 1) Against a waist-level stable object; 2) On your knees; 3) On the floor.

➤ **Plank**
Start in the true plank position, the weight of your body resting on your elbows and toes, using core tension to keep your body straight. As you reach failure, drop to your knees. Keep core tension for the remainder of the set.

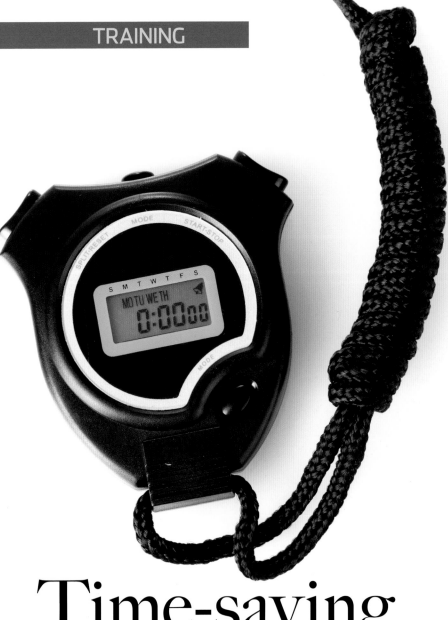

Time-saving Workouts

Tight on time and can't attack one of the main days of the program? These three ultra-efficient routines will work every muscle in your body, while the tough cardio component burns fat long after you've put down the weights.

Time-saving Workout No. 1

Set a timer for 20 minutes. Perform 12 reps of each of the following exercises without resting between them. Record the total number of rounds you perform for future reference. Try to beat your score the next time you do the workout.

EXERCISE
Pushup
Lat Pulldown
Bodyweight Squat
Hammer Curl
Cable Rope Pressdown
Walking Lunge
Lateral Raise
Situp

Time-saving Workout No. 2

Perform the following exercises for 10 complete rounds. Record your total time for future reference. Try to beat your time the next time you do the workout.

EXERCISE	REPS
Deadlift*	5
Stair Climb	60 seconds

*Pick a weight you could do 8–10 reps with. Doing 10 rounds of 5 reps is a lot of deadlifting, so the weight shouldn't be too heavy.

Time-saving Workout No. 3

Set a timer for 10 minutes and complete the following exercises as a continuous circuit with as little rest as possible throughout. Write down how many circuits you're able to complete in the time limit for future reference. Try to beat your score on subsequent attempts.

EXERCISE	REPS
Bodyweight Squat	20
Pushup	15
Lat Pulldown	10

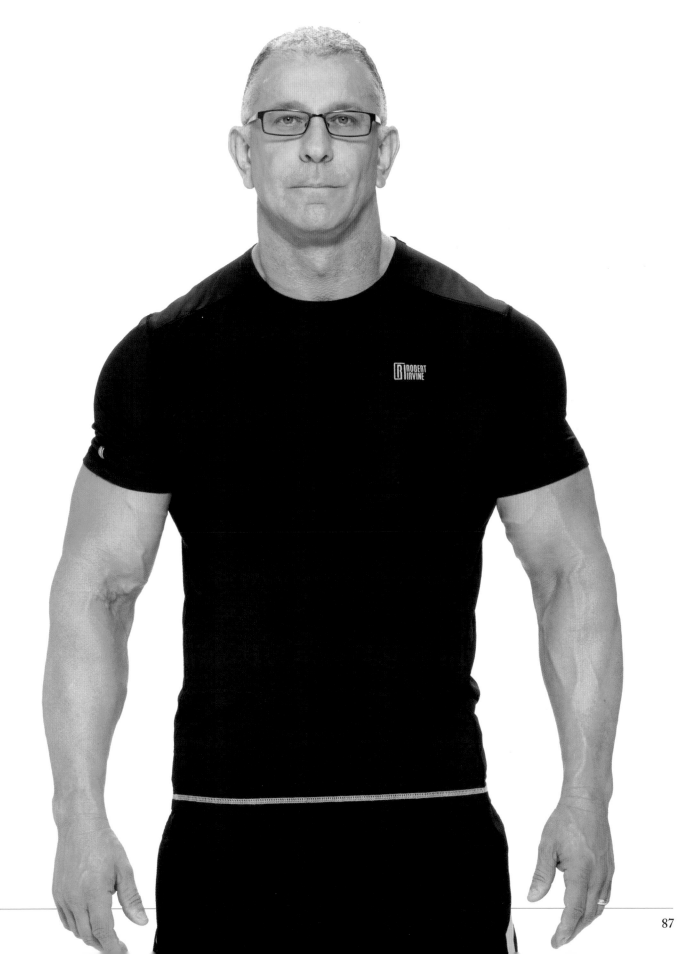

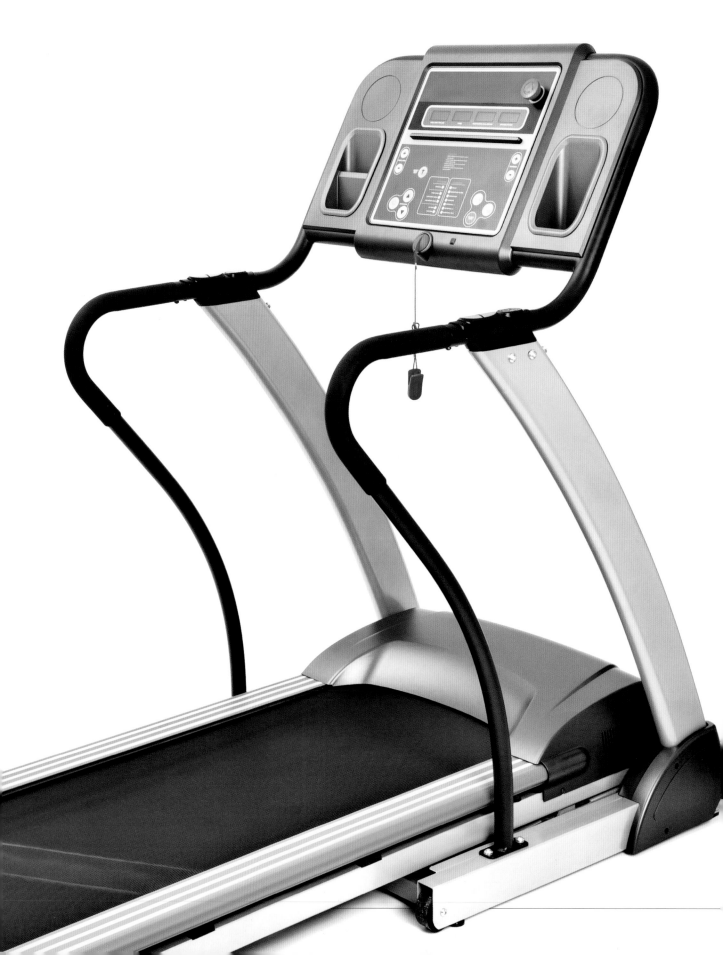

Cardio

Each day's cardio is expressed as a percentage of maximum heart rate, or MHR. We can't say for certain what anyone's safe maximum heart rate is, but exercise scientists theorize that the best way to approximate it is to start with the number 220, then subtract your age. The resulting number represents your MHR.

➤ Maximum Heart Rate (MHR) Calculator

220 – Age = MHR

So, for a 40-year-old person, the calculation would look like this:

220 – 40 = 180 (this person's MHR)

But to play it safe, when you work out, I never want you to hit 100% of your MHR. In each of your cardio sessions, I want you to aim at staying at 65%–75% or 70%–80% of your max heart rate (easily measured on most cardio machines or with a wearable heart-rate monitor).

To figure out what 65%–75% of your MHR would be, let's take the same example of the 40-year-old, who has a 180 MHR. We'll multiply that 180 by the two percentages of the desired range, 65% and 75%, so it will look like this:

180 x .65 = 117 Beats Per Minute (BPM)
180 x .75 = 135 Beats Per Minute (BPM)

So, to stay within 65%–75% of his maximum heart rate, this person's target range would be 117–135 BPM.

Note: When you're ready for High Intensity Interval Training, or HIIT, as explained in the next few paragraphs, don't exceed 85%–90% of your MHR.

HIIT ME: ADVANCED CARDIO

High Intensity Interval Training, or HIIT, is touted by many experts as the ideal way to shed fat and preserve muscle. It involves bursts of intense activity followed by lighter activity—for example, a 20-second sprint followed by a 20-, 30-, or 40-second jog, repeated for a set time.

I've found HIIT to be tremendously helpful in my own training, and encourage you to try it when you feel ready. Steady-state cardio (where your heart rate is elevated but steady) is great for burning calories, and is ideal for beginners; but over time, that calorie burning can make it harder to build or hold on to muscle. For an extreme example of this, compare the bodies of ultramarathoners and track and field sprinters. The former are emaciated; the latter have abundant lean muscle.

My only concern over HIIT is one of readiness. This is an intense form of exercise, and it can wipe you out if your body isn't prepared. Since HIIT sessions tend to drive heart rate higher than my steady-state recommendation, I suggest you start slowly. When you're ready, replace one steady-state cardio session in the workout with 5 minutes of 20-second sprints followed by 40-second jogs on any cardio machine (treadmill, elliptical, bike, rower) or, of course, outside. Once you can do 5 minutes fairly easily, raise the time to 7 minutes, then 10. From there, you can keep increasing total time or whittling away at recovery periods: e.g., sprint for 20 seconds and jog for only 30, working down to a 1:1 work:rest ratio.

In the end, variety is the key not just to keeping your body moving in the right direction, but to keeping your mind stimulated and challenged. Workouts should never feel like they're on autopilot.

So make things hard on yourself. I don't want your workouts to get easier. I just want you to get stronger.

Sample HIIT Session

After a 5- to 10-minute steady-state warmup, set a timer for 10 minutes.

Every minute on the minute, do the following:

➤ **Sprint**
20 seconds

➤ **Jog**
40 seconds

When you finish, do a 5- to 10-minute cooldown.

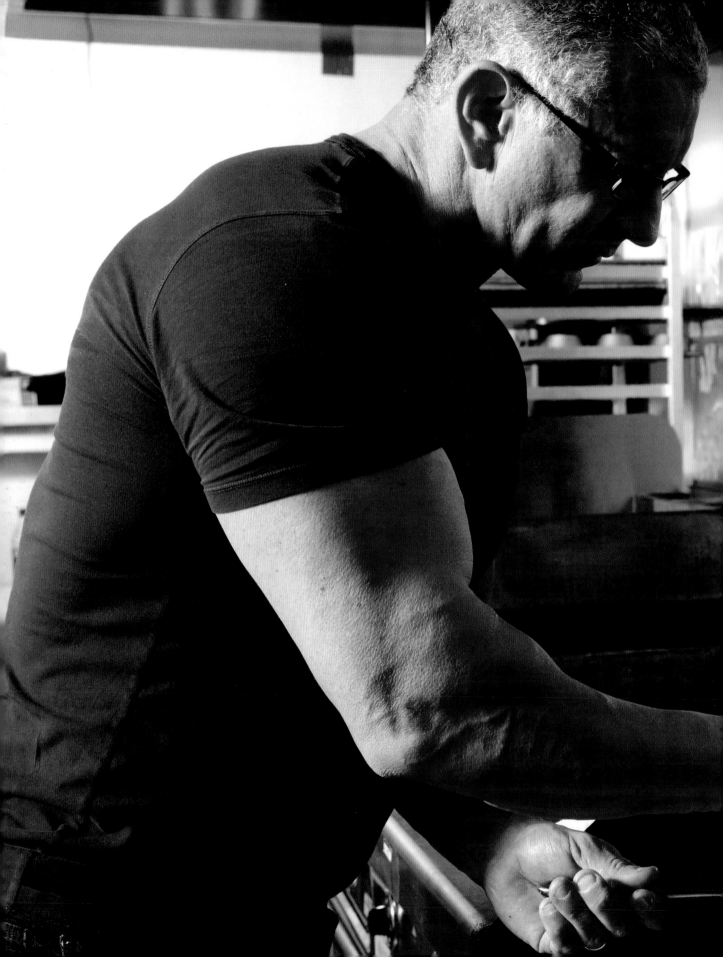

FIT FUEL | **PART III**

Nutrition

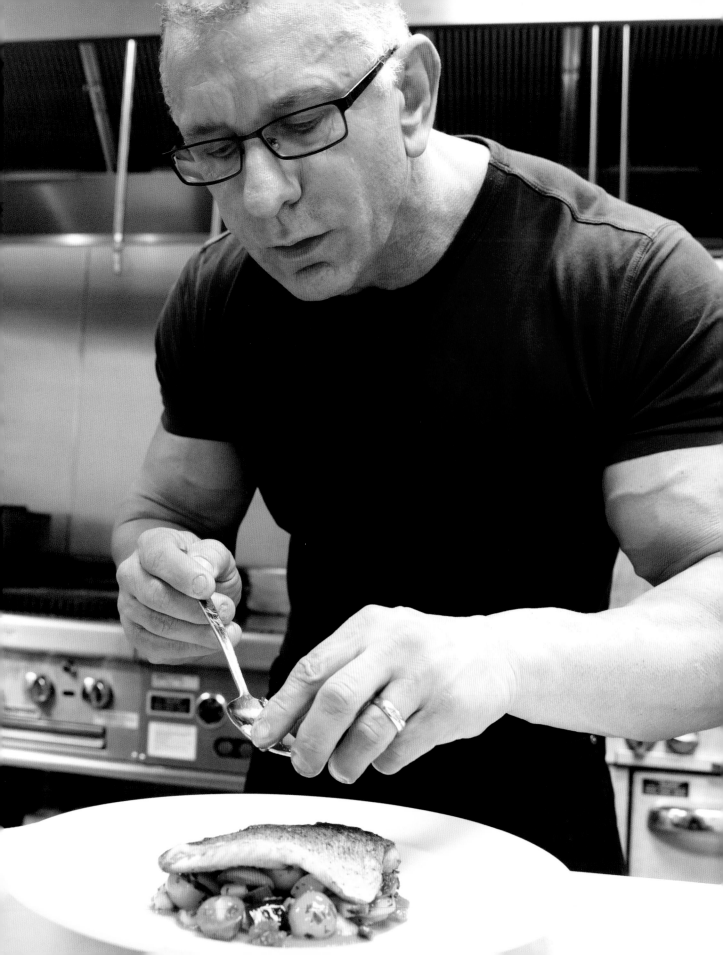

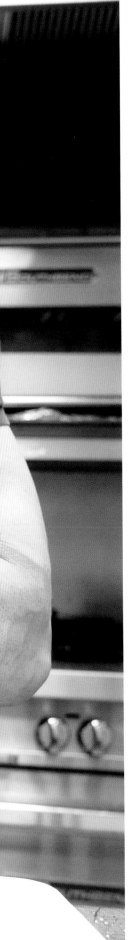

Eat Great and Get in Shape

EATING ISN'T HALF THE BATTLE. I learned the hard way that it's more like 80 percent of the battle. And if so much of your success depends on how you eat, it stands to reason you'd want to not only eat the right things, but also find a way to truly enjoy them. No wonder so many dieters fail when they try to adopt the habits of fitness competitors. If you went from eating bacon, egg, and cheese sandwiches every morning to eating plain oatmeal, you'd be miserable. My entire philosophy is based around making what you need to eat exactly what you'd *want* to eat.

Great Eating: The Principles

1 CONCENTRATE MORE ON WHAT YOU *DO* EAT THAN WHAT YOU DON'T

Most fitness programs and diets are designed and marketed in one of two ways: They're presented as either easy and fun, causing minimal or no disruption to your daily life and existing habits, or as so super-hardcore that merely purchasing them is a major step toward maximizing your potential. That's how most advertisers see you—as either lazy and unable to handle the truth, or as so consumed by fitness that the idea of dying while exercising sounds cool.

I haven't come across too many fitness products or schemes aimed at me and the millions like me—that is, those of us who love both a good workout and a real meal, and who can be categorized as neither lazy nor obsessed. The very idea that you could be perfectly healthy and fit and still enjoy a hearty meal with a glass of red wine or a beer is alien to marketers, so we wind up with the fitness industry we have today: a world of polar extremes.

Meanwhile, most people live somewhere in the middle. I know I do.

Most of us want to be able to enjoy a Fourth of July barbecue without measuring portion sizes on a food scale; to end a big Thanksgiving dinner with a slice of apple pie à la mode with-

out feeling guilty. But we *also* want to be able to look back at the photos from these events and not feel embarrassed about our appearance. We don't want to have to police our friends' Facebook pages and untag ourselves because we look like we're spilling out of our clothes or have a double chin.

As most of us inhabit this middle ground, it should come as no surprise that this is where the answer lies as well.

If you've been even remotely paying attention to the news over the past 15 years, you know that eating fast food regularly is a sure path to obesity and chronic illness. You've probably also learned that you need to stay away from trans fats, in the form of hydrogenated oils, at all costs because the body has an incredibly difficult time breaking them down. So you avoid McDonald's and Burger King, and don't fill your shopping cart with Doritos and Oreos... yet you're still fat and out of shape—and exasperated by the state of your life.

Before you can move forward, you need to understand that simply avoiding obviously bad foods is only a small part of eating for health and fitness. The eating philosophy that's going to get you to your goal is much more about centering every meal around nutrient-dense

+ TIP SHEET

Learn to appreciate and even love the process of cooking. The more you care about what you're doing, the more the fruits of your labor will pay you back.

whole foods prepared with minimal added fat, sugar, and salt.

That may sound like a simple statement, but it's much easier said than done. Once you make the change a part of your life, however, it will feel natural.

2 DON'T WAIT FOR THE "RIGHT TIME" TO EAT RIGHT—THERE WILL NEVER BE ONE!

Likewise, one of the biggest mistakes people make is adopting an all-or-nothing mentality when it comes to healthy eating.

A classic example of this is a scenario I see play out all the time: You start a new diet and exercise regimen on a Monday, follow it to the letter all week, go out with your friends on a Saturday night planning to eat healthy, then have one too many drinks—and before you know it you're stumbling into a Taco Bell at two in the morning.

And instead of getting right back on track with your diet, you throw up your hands and say, "Oh, well, what's the difference? I'll just hang out and eat whatever I want today, then get back to being healthy tomorrow."

Now, if it were truly just a day or a night that you were going off the track, it really wouldn't be so bad. A single day of eating like crap isn't going to make you obese, just as a single day of eating well and training hard isn't going to get you into shape.

But the problem with caving in and saying you'll get back on track tomorrow is that the cycle is destined to repeat itself. Submit to it once, and every social function that arises where the drinks are flowing and the hors d'oeuvres are piled high becomes an open invite to eat like shit and set your goals aside. Before you know it you're riding this diet-and-exercise/bad-food-and-alcohol roller coaster all year long; then when the plates of Christmas cookies are everywhere you look in December, you say to yourself, "I'll just get back at it in January." That's a whole year of your life riddled with anxiety because tomorrow is always the day you'll start.

You have to shake off the notion that the time is ever going to be just right for you to get started. Life doesn't offer many perfect moments—it's complicated and busy, full of unexpected turns, distractions, and setbacks. The idea that you're going to wake up one day and it'll be the perfect day to start eating healthy and training hard is a fallacy. It will never "just happen." You have to make it happen through consistent effort. You have to understand that in the beginning, especially if you're coming at this completely fresh, it's going to suck. There's no easier or quicker way, so stop looking for one. Stop talking about it, stop thinking about it, and stop procrastinating.

It's time to get on with the hard work of getting in the best shape of your life.

3 BUY LOCAL WHEN YOU CAN— THE PAYOFF CAN BE HUGE

If there's a good local market near you where you can buy everything you need, great. But even if you can get only a few items like veggies and herbs at a local farm stand, it's worth the trip. Nine times out of 10, the food you get there is going to be fresher, treated with fewer pesticides, and—since it spent less time in a storage house waiting to move halfway around the country (or the world)—it'll be more nutrient-dense, and therefore much healthier.

The longer it sits in some warehouse, the more food deteriorates, the fewer nutrients it has, and the less it's worth to your body, to say nothing of your taste buds.

4 BEWARE FOOD-LABEL BOMBS THAT COULD BLOW UP IN YOUR FACE

"Low-fat," "organic," "natural," "grass-fed," "humane"… Understanding the oftentimes baffling terminology on food labels can be one of the most frustrating aspects of trying to eat for health and fitness. But it's worth the trouble to learn what these terms mean, since they can so greatly affect both your nutritional intake and your fitness goals.

There's also the fact that, even if a food is labeled "natural and organic," it can still wreak havoc. You can have "natural, organic" cakes, pies, and chips, but do you really need me to tell you that brownies marked "organic" will make you just as fat as the ones from Sara Lee? Organic sugar will plump you up the same way high-fructose corn syrup will. Ditto organic butter and white flour.

On page 96, I break down the label terms you're most likely to come across. Familiarize yourself with them before the next time you go food shopping.

5 IF YOU CAN'T PRONOUNCE IT, DON'T EAT IT

Look at the ingredient label of any processed food item and you'll be overwhelmed by the number of unpronounceable flavorings and preservatives it contains, most or all of which were formulated in a petri dish in some lab. Michael Pollan, author of one of the best books ever written about nutrition, *Food Rules*, famously said that if you can't easily pronounce an ingredient, don't eat the food it's in.

It's a great rule to follow no matter what kinds of foods you like to eat or what your dietary goals are. Though the ramifications of making such a decision are significant: Strictly following this principle would eliminate virtually all processed foods from your diet.

So, why bother?

Pollan and other experts in the field theorize that the human body hasn't evolved to the

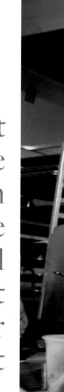

You must shake the notion that the time will be just right for you to get started.

point where it can break down all these complex chemical formulations and digest them easily. If you don't follow this rule 100 percent of the time, are you in trouble? No. But the more often you can follow it, the better.

6 CALL JUNK FOOD WHAT IT IS: A DRUG CREATED TO ADDICT YOU

Aside from ingredients your body can't easily process, there's something even more sinister afoot, says investigative reporter Michael Moss.

As he chronicles in his book *Salt Sugar Fat: How the Food Giants Hooked Us*, many processed foods have been specifically designed by the major food companies to get us hooked on them so we'll eat more of them. Moss describes

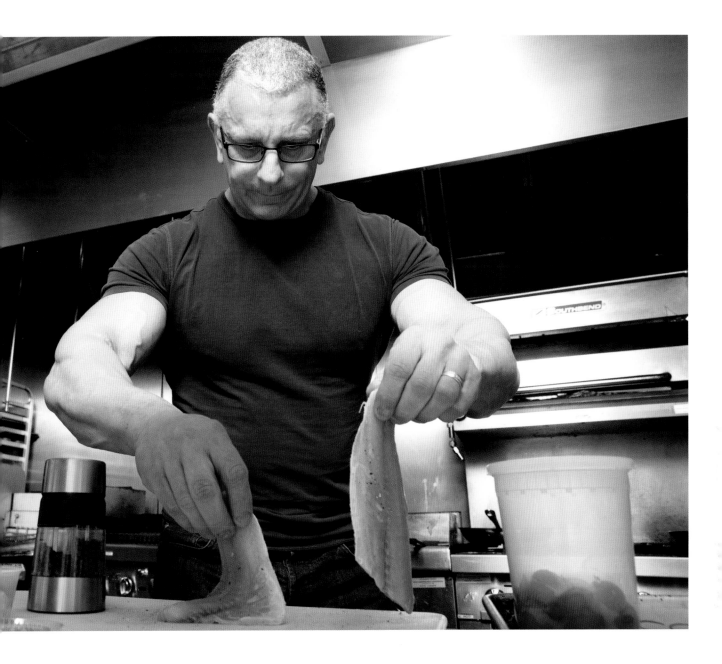

how the salty, fatty, crunchy taste of the most popular snack chips isn't based on a recipe that was stumbled upon by accident in someone's kitchen. It was fine-tuned in a laboratory to trick our bodies into craving these "treats"—and, consequently, us into buying huge amounts of them, resulting in record profits for the processed-food industry (not to mention sky-rocketing obesity rates).

Being armed with that knowledge, why take a chance on eating this junk? If one day at work when you're starving and don't have time for a meal you grab a single-serve bag of chips from the vending machine, will you automatically lose all your hard work in the gym? No. But a nutritionally empty bag of chips can do more

damage than the sum of its calories. For many people it will do exactly what it was designed to do: act as a trigger to get you to eat more, so eventually you find yourself saying, "Oh, screw it!" and throwing your whole healthy eating plan out the window for that day.

Don't take the risk. Eliminate these trigger foods from your diet, and replace them with healthy, home-cooked meals.

7 DON'T BUY YOUR CHEAT FOODS AHEAD OF TIME

Cheats play a key role in any sustainable diet—they keep you sane and, when timed right (like on hard training days), keep your metabolism cranked up high. But their role is limited.

When you're at the store buying the week's groceries, that's not the time to be planning ahead for your cheat meal. Deciding on your cheat day that you want ice cream and going to an ice cream parlor for a treat is far better than putting a half-gallon container of ice cream in your cart while you're shopping, thinking you'll save it for later in the week.

The temptation of having junk food around is often too difficult to resist even for the most dedicated athletes and fitness models, so most have learned to never have the crap in the house in the first place. Keeping a store of cookies and chips in your cabinet is a disaster waiting to happen. It turns your kitchen into a minefield.

Make it simple: Don't buy it.

Food Labels: A Basic Primer

"LOW-FAT" Contains 3 grams of fat or less for a given serving size.

BOTTOM LINE It's all in the serving size. If you buy a packet of three "low-fat" cookies and the serving size is one cookie, the problem is self-evident: You're at risk of eating all three, tripling your serving size and the amount of fat (and simple carbs) you consume. The low-fat label is also beside the point. Fat isn't the enemy—overindulging is.

"ORGANIC" Foods with the "organic" label must be raised or grown following methods deemed acceptable by the USDA. The fertilizer/feed for crops or herds must not use synthetic products or genetic engineering. Foods bearing this label must be 95 percent organic or more.

BOTTOM LINE You don't need to clean out your fridge and cupboard and buy only organic foods, but it does pay to buy organic meat and dairy, which can have higher levels of heart-healthy omega-3 fatty acids. Plus, when you buy regular meat and dairy, you may wind up ingesting more of a compound called insulin-like growth factor (IGF-1), which has been linked to cancer. Nonorganic produce will also have had more exposure to pesticides. With fruits like bananas and oranges, which have thick, inedible peels, this is less of a factor; but fruit like apples, pears, and peaches, with their thin, edible skins, are more susceptible to absorbing pesticides.

"NATURAL" This label means a food was "minimally" processed and contains no artificial ingredients. Shockingly, a food can still be labeled "natural" and have been subjected to hormones and antibiotics. The natural label can be applied only to meat and eggs.

BOTTOM LINE The natural label adds little nutritional value to the food. It's neither particularly good nor misleading, so you'll need to look beyond it to what else is in the food to make an informed decision.

"FREE-RANGE" AND "CAGE-FREE" These aren't as animal-friendly as they sound. With both labels, the indoor space animals inhabit most of their lives could still be cramped and filthy; the difference regards only outdoor space. Free-range animals are raised with access to an outdoor area—not necessarily the case with those labeled cage-free. And remember, just because it's "outdoors" doesn't mean it's a pleasant place to be.

BOTTOM LINE Cage-free doesn't mean much for the health of the animal, and free-range is only slightly better. Try to keep an eye out for the far less ubiquitous label "pasture-raised"—according to the USDA, a pasture-raised animal must have "continuous and unconfined access to pasture throughout their life cycle."

"HUMANE" Some farms that claim their animals are raised "humanely" might be telling the truth, some might not. There are no set USDA regulations certifying what humane actually is.

BOTTOM LINE If it's important to you that animals are raised humanely, get to know your local farmers, or look for the Certified Humane label, which is independently verified by the nonprofit Humane Farm Animal Care organization.

"GRASS-FED" Animals from which "grass-fed" meat comes may still have had part of their diet supplemented with grains. Look for meat labeled "100% grass-fed" or "pasture-raised."

BOTTOM LINE This is an important label because cattle raised on grain provide meat that contains fewer omega-3 and more omega-6 fats. While omega-6 fats are not, in and of themselves, unhealthy, the amount of them found in the modern diet is. Americans tend to eat 11–30 times more omega-6 than omega-3 fats, which researchers theorize could be a significant factor in the rising number of inflammatory disorders. Grass-fed meat flips this ratio, giving you more omega-3s than omega-6s.

"NO ANTIBIOTICS"/"ANTIBIOTIC-FREE" Many animals are given antibiotics in order to fight the infections they'll likely contract in an unclean living environment. When animals become resistant to these drugs, however, they can still carry bacteria—which you might ingest if you undercook your meat. It's hard to trace particular instances of the phenomenon, but some cases of food poisoning might be attributed to meat from antibiotic-resistant animals.

BOTTOM LINE Antibiotics have become a necessity at some factory farms due to unsanitary conditions. Looking for this label can take you another step away from inhumane practices and unhealthy food products.

"NO ADDED HORMONES" Federal regulations don't technically allow farmers to administer hormones or steroids to poultry, pigs, or goats (cattle are the exception), but it's hard to say how many farmers actually comply.

BOTTOM LINE Knowing your farmer is the only way to be certain your meat is hormone-free.

"NON-GMO" Referring to genetically modified organisms, this label ensures that none of the food's ingredients contain anything that was altered at the gene level.

BOTTOM LINE I'm not sold that GMO foods are inherently bad for you or otherwise dangerous to the environment. However, I do think it's wise to err on the side of filling your diet with as many whole, natural foods as possible. So "non-GMO" is not the be-all and end-all label, but I believe it does add value to what you're buying.

"GLUTEN-FREE" Foods with this label need to contain less than 20 parts per million of gluten. Gluten is the protein in a grain of wheat, barley, and rye, which, among other things, gives bread, rolls, and wraps a chewy texture. Celiac disease, which affects about one in 100 people, is an autoimmune disorder that causes the body to attack the small intestine when gluten is ingested.

BOTTOM LINE Though Celiac disease is not common, gluten-free diets have gone mainstream, with many people who don't suffer from Celiac disease reporting great success. This isn't a huge surprise, since gluten-free diets restrict processed carbohydrates. Again, I'd urge you not to demonize a particular food, especially one you love, in the name of getting fit. This might lead to cravings that can get out of control. Limit bread and processed carbs, certainly, but never say never.

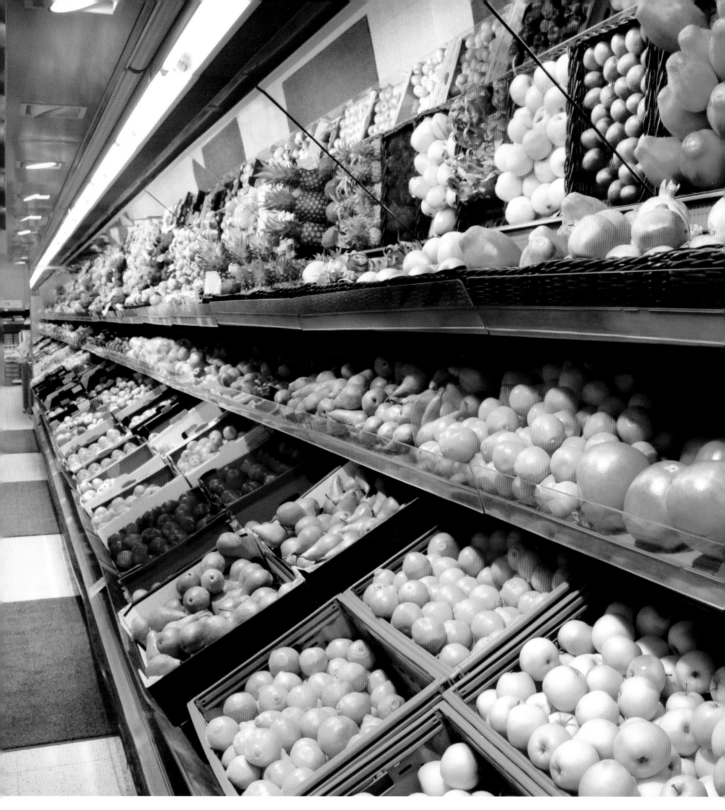

Fruit is a great option, but easy to overdo. Try to limit fruit intake to one or two pieces per day, or to the 60-minute post-workout window, when your depleted muscles will use it to refuel.

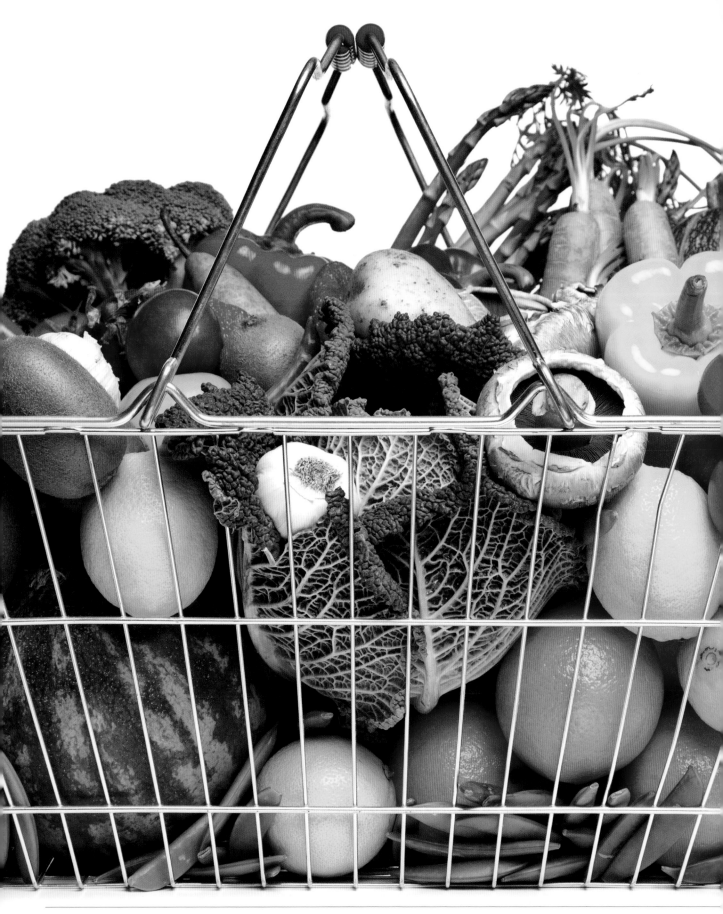

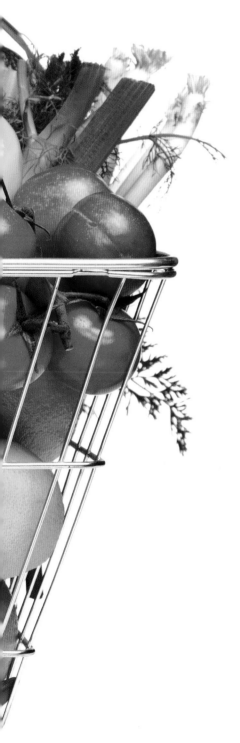

Great Eating: The Shopping List

IT ALL STARTS IN THE SUPERMARKET. This is your armory, the place you go to load up your battle gear. Shop well and you set yourself up for success. Shop poorly, and you've got no chance to win. I've broken my shopping list down into 10 must-haves. They are:

1 VEGGIES
2 VEGGIES
3 MORE VEGGIES!

This looks like overkill, but trust me, it's not. As soon as you get your grocery cart, the produce section should be the first place you go. Any diet that limits vegetable intake is just a faster way to die. You might lose weight on the way, but you won't be around long to enjoy it.

Especially with regard to fibrous vegetables such as broccoli, cauliflower, spinach, kale, and the like—eat as much as you want, whenever you want. These should line the bottom of your grocery cart. They're nutrient-dense, they fill you up, and they promote intestinal motility—which is just a fancy way of saying that they're going to keep you nice and regular. It might not be polite talk, but I know everyone appreciates that!

+ TIP SHEET
Vegetables should form the foundation of any healthy diet. If you're eating a lot of vegetables, you're guaranteed to have more energy—and less room in your belly for junk.

4 LEAN PROTEIN

Your fridge should always be well-stocked with chicken and turkey breast, fish (frozen or, if you intend to eat it the same day, fresh), and the occasional piece of lean beef.

Even if you don't have time to cook any of the dishes from the recipe section of this book, it takes a ridiculously short amount of time to steam those vegetables you loaded your cart with (add a little water to a pot over medium-high heat and check them every few minutes to desired tenderness) while you put some grapeseed oil in a pan and sauté a few pieces of chicken with some nice, spicy sriracha.

5 CLEAN CARBS

These include brown and white rice (white for post-workout meals, brown for other meals), sweet potatoes, white potatoes, quinoa, and farro—all foods that are incredibly versatile and can be easily, creatively, and deliciously spruced up.

6 (SOME) HEALTHY FATS

I'm happy to see that healthy dietary fats have gotten a big push in the media in recent years; but even healthy fats like nuts and avocado require moderation. As noted in the section about macros on page 104, one gram of protein contains four calories, the same as a gram of carbs. Fat is more than twice as calorically dense as the other macros, with nine calories per gram.

Extra-virgin olive oil is great, of course, but its low smoking point can make it tough to cook with in some instances. Take a look through the recipe section and you'll notice that you're not going to be able to make very many of my recipes without grapeseed oil, an unfortunately overlooked healthy fat with a high smoking point (especially compared to olive oil).

7 (SOME) FRUIT

Again, why only some? As with fat, eating too much fruit is easy to do. I don't want you to be scared of fruit, since it's completely unprocessed, convenient, and nutrient-dense. But at the same time, you should limit your intake to one or two pieces per day. Simple carbs spike insulin, which drives nutrients to muscle and fat cells. The insulin spike you might get from the fast-digesting carbs of an apple, orange, or banana are mitigated by fiber, but it's still easy to overdo.

For maximum benefit, limit your fruit intake to post-workout meals. The sugars will refuel glycogen stores and halt the breakdown of muscle tissue—meaning, they'll have less chance of being stored as fat.

8 HOT SAUCE

I put sriracha sauce on everything. For clean eating it's an absolute lifesaver, as it adds a wonderfully rich flavor, has a nice amount of heat that's tolerable for the average person, and aids digestion (since chili peppers and vinegar are the two main ingredients, and vinegar may help break down food in your stomach).

Of course, sriracha isn't the only sauce that works. Tabasco sauce, Cholula hot sauce, and Frank's RedHot are all pretty good. Try a variety and see which fit your particular tastes.

9 KOSHER OR SEA SALT

The salt shaker on your kitchen table is probably filled with iodized salt. I'm not a fan of table salt because of the extensive refining it undergoes, which strips it of minerals.

Plus, iodized salt has aluminum compounds added to it to prevent clumping, which in large quantities may cause neurological disorders—and having salt that falls easily out of the shaker doesn't seem like a fair trade-off for ingesting potentially damaging substances, no matter how minuscule the amount.

Kosher salt and sea salt don't have this problem, and they're a lot tastier, too.

And, finally, one essential nonfood for your list:

10 REUSABLE FOOD-STORAGE CONTAINERS

This one is straight out of the bodybuilders' playbook. Don't worry, I'm not going to tell you to buy a bucket of fake tanner, too; but there's a lot to be said for how disciplined these men and women are when it comes to preparing food ahead of time so they're never without a healthy meal.

How many times have you succumbed to eating the same crap everyone else around you is eating because you were starving? It's really not that difficult (or strange) to load up a portable container with a meal to take with you for the day. There's nothing sadder than starting the morning with good intentions, eating a healthy breakfast, then going out for the day, losing track of time, and winding up eating some fast-food garbage because you ran out of options.

If you're really going to make a lasting change, these moments can't happen.

The great thing about eating my way: Once you start doing it, you're not going to want to eat any other way. This food satisfies you and gives you energy rather than sapping it.

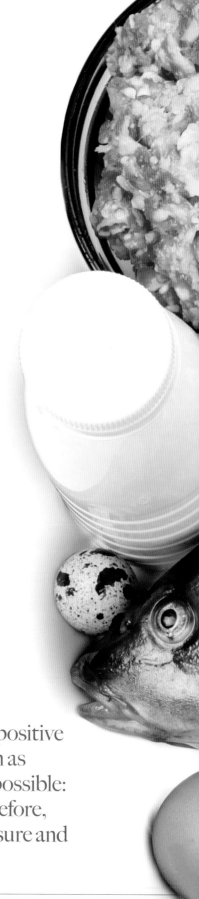

I've experienced firsthand the positive effects of a diet that's filled with as many whole, natural foods as possible: I have more energy than ever before, and I've kicked the blood-pressure and cholesterol medications.

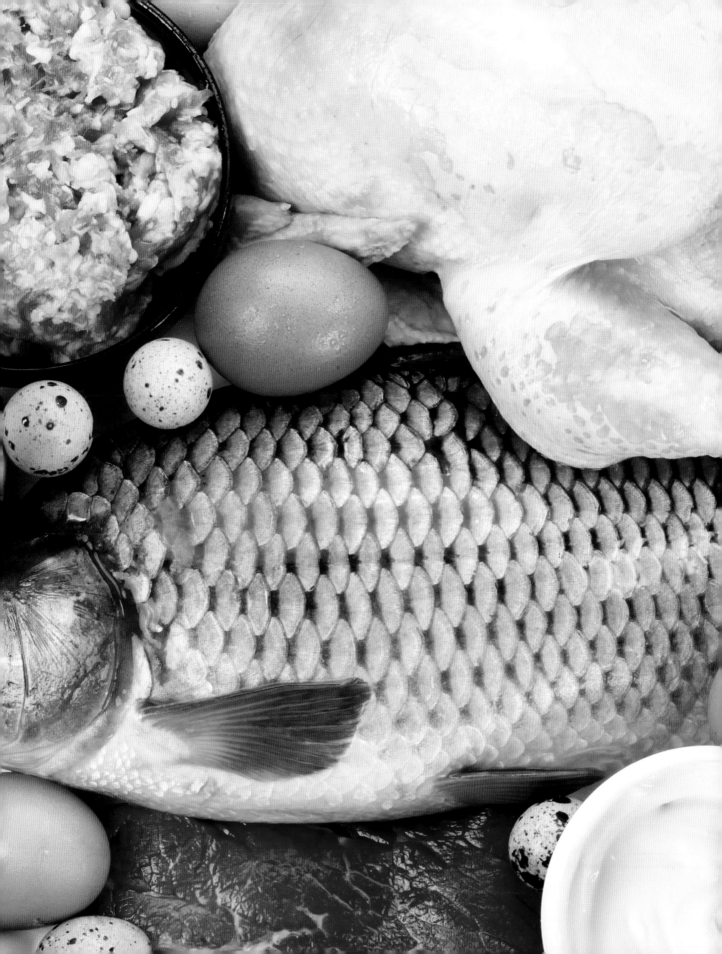

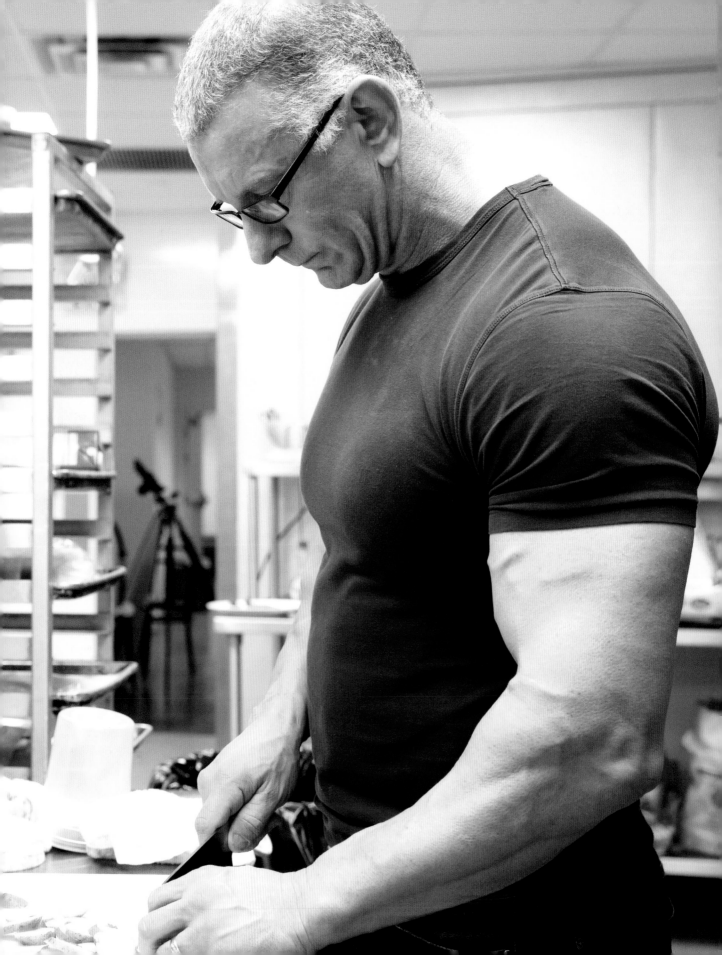

My Favorite Ingredients

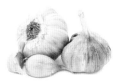

➤ THROUGHOUT THE RECIPE SECTION of this book, you're going to come across some recurring ingredients. These ingredients didn't become my go-tos for no reason—in all instances there are terrific health benefits to be derived from using them on a regular basis. Here are a few of my favorite ingredients to incorporate regularly, along with the reasons I consider them indispensable.

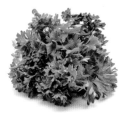

GRAPESEED OIL

Why It has a high smoking point of 420°, which makes it the perfect oil to fry with. It also contains linoleic acid, a healthy polyunsaturated fat that can help fight LDL (bad) cholesterol.

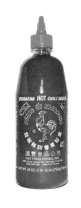

SRIRACHA

Why The initial burning sensation you feel when it hits your tongue turns into a pleasurable release of endorphins in just a few minutes. And it's made of capsaicin, which can help speed up metabolism, improve blood flow by dissolving blood clots, and fight inflammation.

QUINOA

Why One of the few complete plant proteins, quinoa has all the essential amino acids needed to initiate protein synthesis; twice the fiber of most other grains; and lysine, an amino acid that aids in muscle repair.

FRISÉE LETTUCE

Why It's an excellent source of roughage (which improves intestinal motility); vitamins A, C, and K; and folate.

PARSLEY

Why Its volatile oils, like myristicin, may blunt the formation of tumors. It's also a natural diuretic, which can help flush excess fluid from the body and improve kidney function. Further, it's an inflammatory fighter, and contains blood-pressure-lowering folic acid.

GARLIC

Why Regularly eating raw garlic can greatly reduce your risk of lung cancer: Subjects in one study reduced their risk of the deadly disease by 44 percent. Garlic can also decrease the frequency of colds.

OLIVES

Why They contain high amounts of vitamin E; plus, their monounsaturated fats can decrease LDL (bad) cholesterol levels and triglycerides while boosting HDL (good) cholesterol, thus lowering the risk of heart attack.

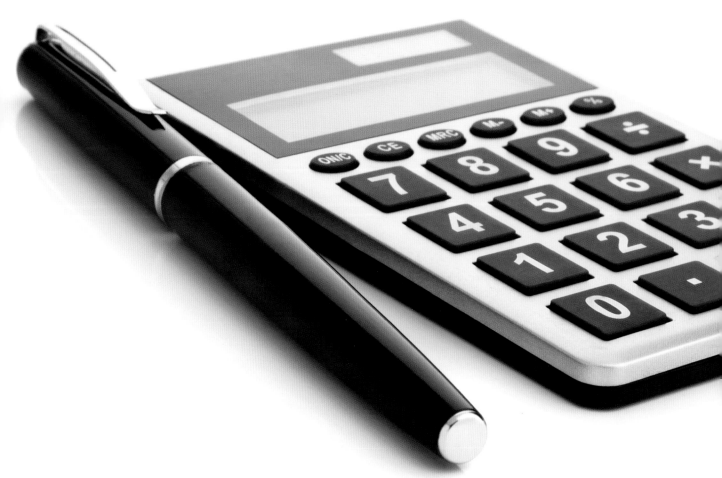

Macros, Calories & How Much You Really Need to Eat

NOW THAT YOU KNOW what foods to buy, the next question is, How much should you actually eat? If you're trying to lose weight, the simple answer is: Eat less than you need. Here, I'll show you how to calculate exactly how much that is.

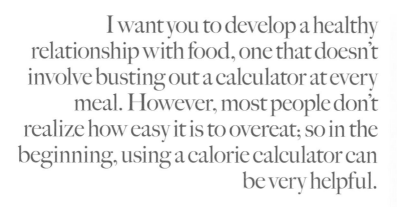

> I want you to develop a healthy relationship with food, one that doesn't involve busting out a calculator at every meal. However, most people don't realize how easy it is to overeat; so in the beginning, using a calorie calculator can be very helpful.

Throughout the recipe section of this book, you'll see a box at the bottom of each recipe listing the value of the "macros," or macronutrients. There are three macronutrients: carbohydrates, fats, and protein.

What do these macros do? In the broadest of strokes, it's fair to say that protein builds and maintains muscle tissue; carbs fuel daily activity; and fat ensures healthy function of a number of organs and bodily processes. But at its base level, all food is merely energy, expressed as calories.

Not all macros deliver the same amount of energy. Each gram of carbohydrate or protein is approximately four calories, while each gram of fat is approximately nine calories, making fat more calorically dense. That's why, when you see that a dish has more protein or carbohydrates than fat, you can't consider that the whole story. It's also why, no matter what your goal, you should eat less fat and more of the other two macronutrients in a given day.

To start losing weight, you'll have to eat less than your body needs to maintain its current weight. If you're in the enviable position of being at a healthy body weight but wanting to gain muscle mass, you'll have to eat more than your body needs, preferably getting the excess calories from lean protein.

Figuring out what your body needs boils down to math, and there are a number of well-established scientific equations you can use. The Mifflin-St. Jeor

Equation is probably the most accurate formula available for calculating resting metabolic rate, or the number of calories your body needs to execute its daily functions. The equation works like this: For men, all you have to do is take the number 10, multiply it by your current body weight in kilograms, add it to the result of your height in centimeters multiplied by 6.25, then subtract the result of your age multiplied by 5. Add 5 to that number and you've got your RMR, or resting metabolic rate. Ladies, instead of adding 5 at the end of the equation, subtract 161. Then, once you've got your RMR, adjust your daily calories to lose (or gain) weight.

See how *easy* and *fun* this is!

OR...

If you've got this new thing called the Internet, head over to *fitfuelbook.com/calc,* type all your information into the calorie calculator, and get your results instantly. The calculator can even account for your current activity levels.

Right—so if you can just type it in online, why did I show you the whole damn thing here? I'm not trying to blind you with science. I did it because I want to show you that losing weight (or gaining it) is really just mathematics. Hit the right number and you win. Miss it and you set yourself back.

Of course, how you spend those calories is important. You'll want to shoot for at least 0.5 grams of protein per pound of body weight per day to maintain muscle mass. (A 200-pound person would need at least 100 grams of protein.) Because building and maintaining muscle mass is so important to your overall health, I recommend erring a bit on the higher side of protein intake, from about 0.7 grams up to 1.2 grams per pound of body weight. You'll get the rest of your calories from about the same amount of carbs and around half the fat, keeping total caloric intake where you need it for your particular goal.

Eventually, as you grow accustomed to eating the right amount, you'll know what to do just by listening to your body. While you're still learning, however, I recommend using a calculator and being mindful of your numbers. You may not realize how many calories you're actually taking in versus how many your body needs till you do the math. Until you get to the point where you can eyeball a serving size, it's all too easy to lie to yourself and think you're eating less than you are.

Numbers, however, don't lie.

What About Supplements?

> The only thing more confusing than the myriad food labels you need to be able to decipher is the huge number of supplements available on the market today. There are some great supplements out there, and I do believe the good ones far outweigh the useless and dangerous ones. To cut through the confusion, I have a rule of three. Meaning, I believe there are three supplements that are safe and effective for just about everyone to take. In order of importance, they are: fish oil, multivitamins, and whey and/or casein protein.

Are these supplements necessary for everyone to take? No. If you're eating a well-balanced diet, you should be fine. However, I can't think of a good reason not to take fish oil—its heart-health benefits are extremely well-documented and very little has been said to contradict these findings. A multivitamin is a great insurance policy against potentially missing any key nutrients in a given day. And a protein supplement, best taken after a workout, makes it easier to hit your protein requirements. If you're a vegetarian or simply find it hard to eat enough protein, then you should definitely consider a supplement.

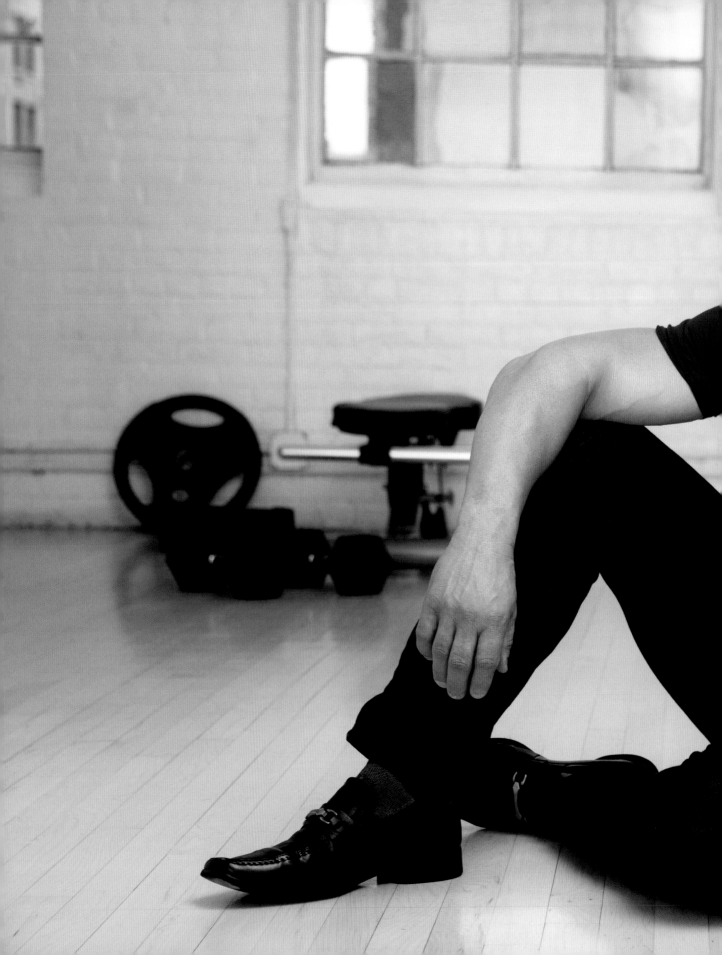

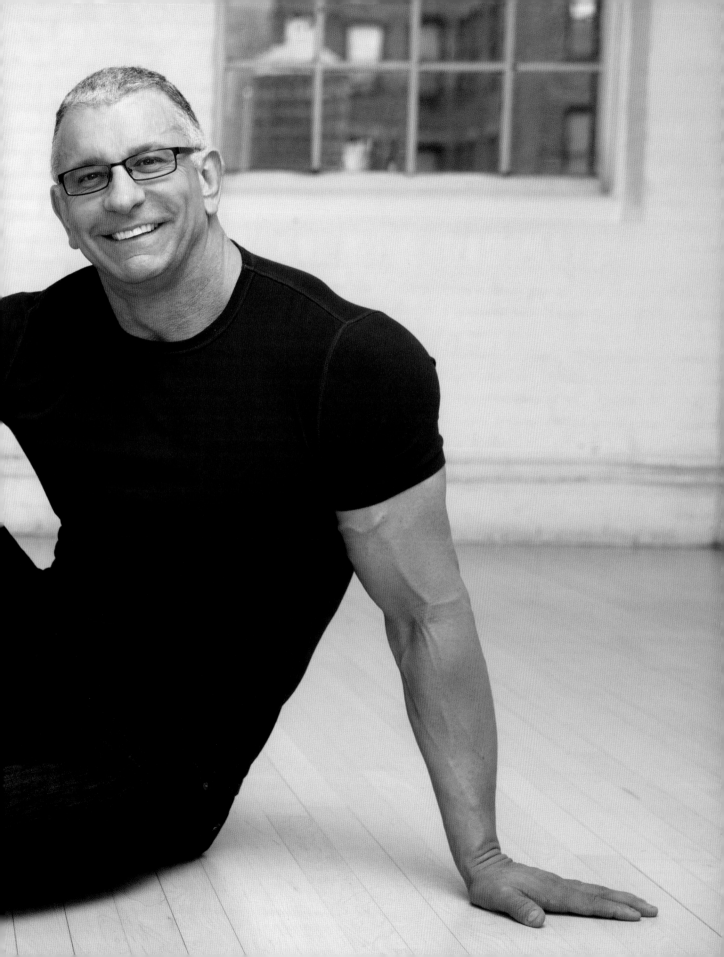

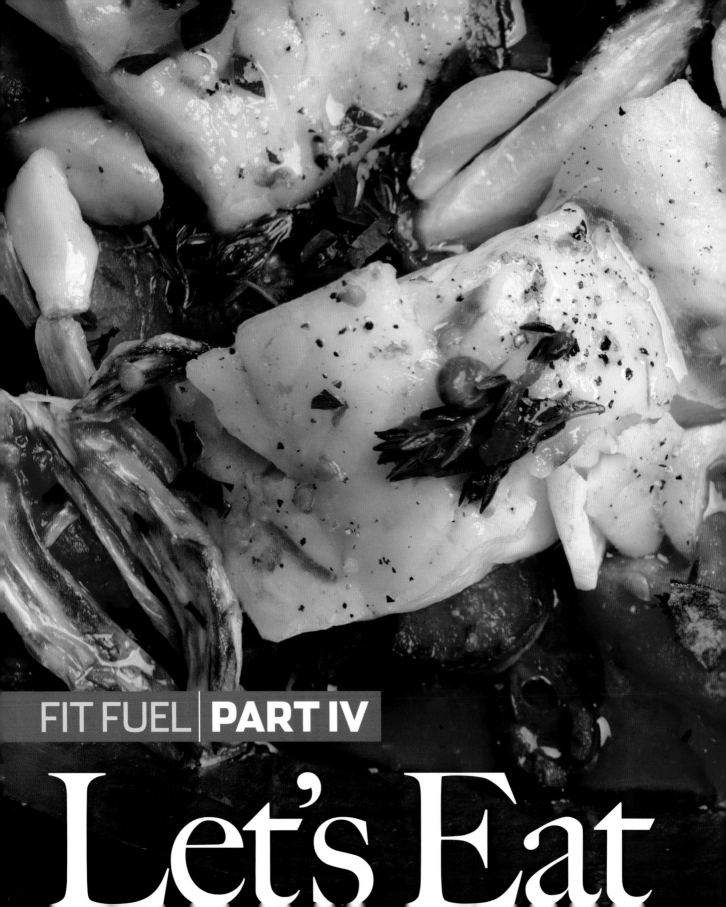

Let's Eat

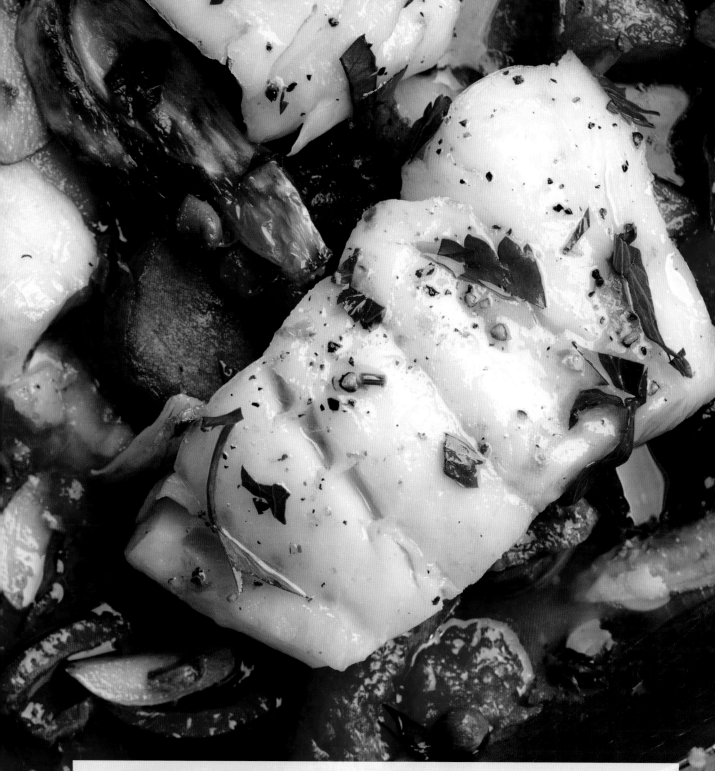

Meal Recommendations

Throughout the recipe section, you'll notice that I've made recommendations next to each recipe, designating a meal as ideal for certain times or days: Any Day; A Post-workout Meal; A Hard Training Day; or A Cheat Day. These are not hard-and-fast rules. In the Nutrition Chapter, I illustrated how weight loss or gain is a matter of total calories consumed. With that said, I've had great success by timing certain meals. For instance, eating high-carb meals after a workout or saving a heavier meal for days when I train particularly hard. You'll eventually figure out what works best for you, but in the beginning, these recommendations will help guide you.

All salt and pepper ingredients are "to taste" unless otherwise noted. I prefer kosher or sea salt in most recipes.

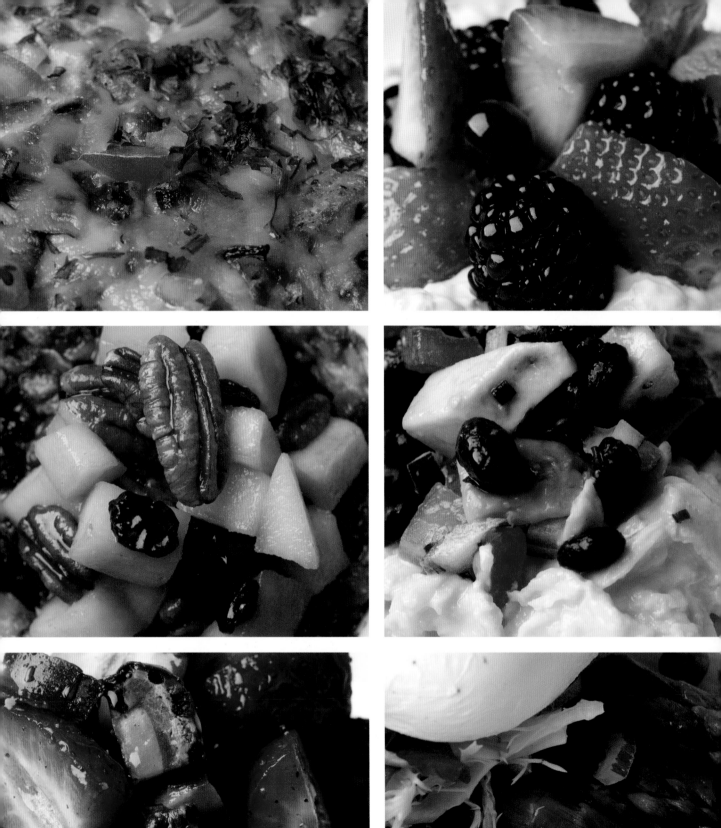

The Menu
Breakfast

Peanut Butter Crunch Protein Pancakes

The classic belly bombs get a makeover in this nutritious yet decadent recipe.

THERE ARE FEW JOYS IN LIFE as simple and wonderful as sitting down with the family on a Sunday morning and enjoying a stack of hot pancakes. But there's a stark difference between growing young boys and girls who possess raging hormones and are literally getting taller by the day, and adults who, well... aren't. Not only doesn't your metabolism work the way it used to, but—and here's another sad truth behind the ubiquitous Sunday-pancake tradition—your body makes no distinction between pure table sugar and the white flour that's the central ingredient of most boxed pancake mixes.

That's where my Peanut Butter Crunch Protein Pancakes come in. With this recipe, not only do we deliver a big shot of protein via chopped pieces of one of my own Fit Crunch protein bars, we also lower the glycemic index of the dish by replacing white flour with a combination of whole-wheat pastry flour and flaxseed meal. Instead of prepackaged maple syrup (most of which is really just high-fructose corn syrup), we top the dish with a combination of sliced strawberries and stevia, a sugar-free plant-based sweetener.

The end result is the decadent, rich, satisfying taste you've come to expect from a pancake breakfast, but with a much better macro profile and myriad health benefits: Each tablespoon of flaxseed meal contains nearly 2 grams of heart-healthy omega-3 fats, plus fiber and lignans, which have been shown to improve prostate health in men and ease menopausal symptoms in women.

Ideal for: A Post-workout Meal
Makes 6 Servings

+ YOU'LL NEED

1½ **cups** low-fat milk

1 **egg**

6 **tbsp** brown flaxseed meal

½ **tsp** salt

3 **tsp** baking powder

2 **tbsp** honey

1½ **cups** whole-wheat pastry flour

1 **tbsp** grapeseed oil

1 Fit Crunch peanut butter protein bar, chopped

12 strawberries, sliced

2 **tbsp** stevia

+ TO MAKE IT

1 In a mixing bowl, stir together milk and egg. Add flaxseed meal, salt, baking powder, honey, and whole-wheat pastry flour until smooth.

2 Heat grapeseed oil in a pan over medium heat, then ladle about ¼ cup mixture into the pan.

3 When bubbles form on top of the cake, sprinkle with pieces of the chopped protein bar.

4 Flip cake and cook until golden brown.

5 Repeat process until all batter has been used.

6 Sprinkle sliced strawberries with stevia and pile on top of pancakes with extra protein bar pieces.

The Macros

268 Calories

11g Protein

8g Fat

39g Carbs

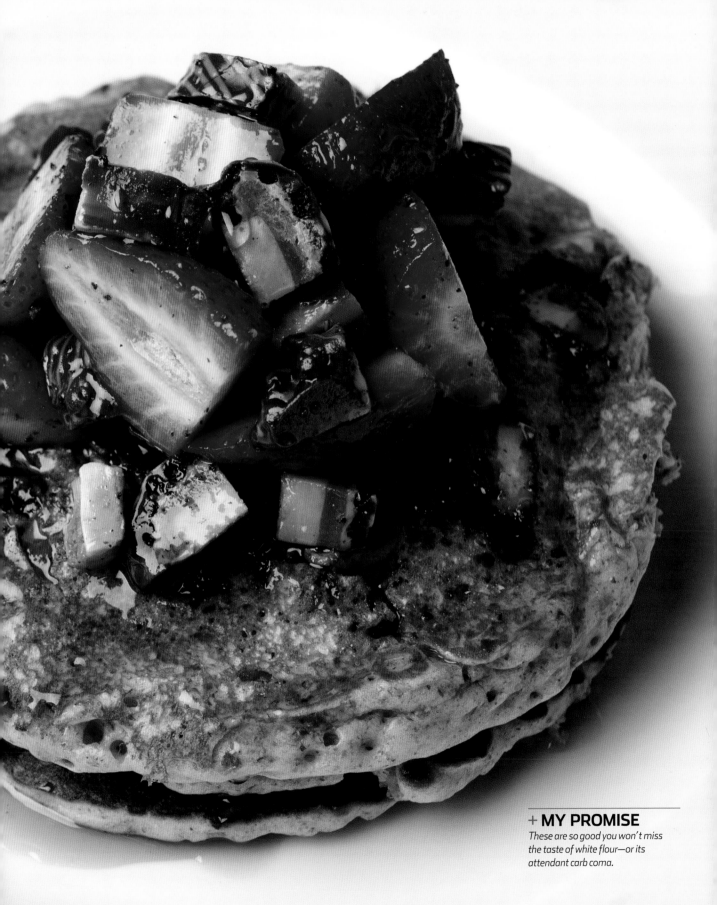

+ MY PROMISE

These are so good you won't miss the taste of white flour—or its attendant carb coma.

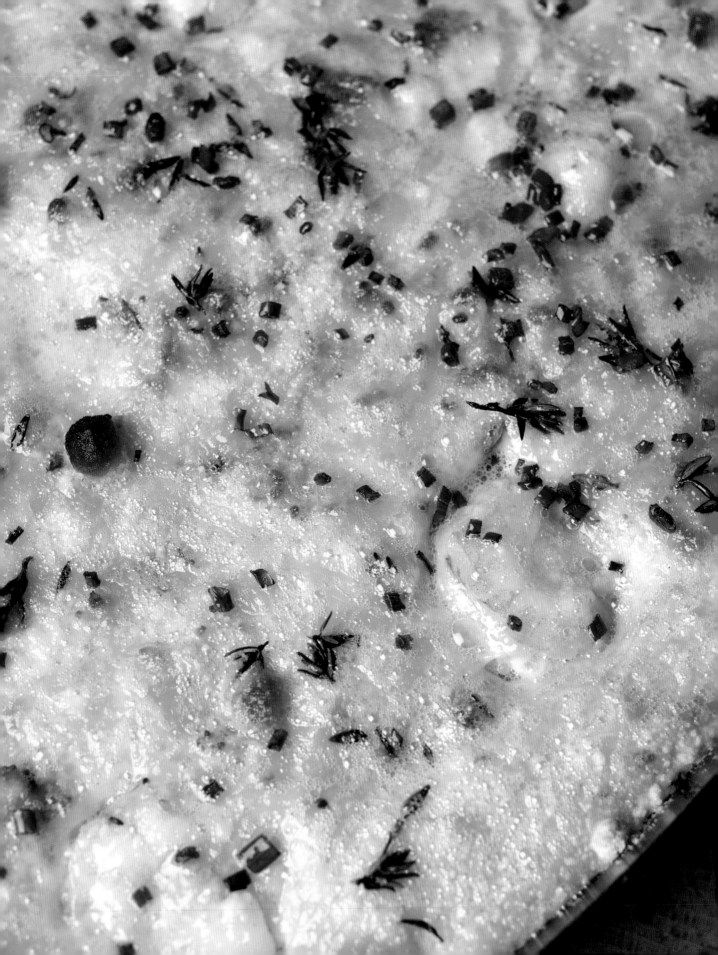

Shrimp &
Leek Polenta Bake

A savory way to start your day.

MOST FOLKS DON'T GET TERRIBLY EXCITED when they hear polenta is on the menu, and it's not hard to see why. Polenta is something of a culinary blank slate, so it really only ever gets as good as the chef who prepares it.

This take on polenta is packed with flavor, and I guarantee that no matter your experience level, you can make this taste like a restaurant-quality effort if you take the time to prep properly.

This Shrimp & Leek Polenta Bake is prepped entirely the night before. All you have to do in the morning is take it out of the fridge, pop it into a preheated oven, and finish it for a minute in the broiler. The end result is a tasty, stick-to-your-ribs meal that's loaded with protein and low-glycemic carbs.

Many of the nutritional benefits of this dish are derived from leeks, known to contain artery-protecting folate as well as kaempferol, a polyphenol that can boost nitric oxide (often referred to as N.O.), which relaxes blood vessels. N.O. also improves blood flow to working muscles while you train.

Breakfast truly is the most important meal of the day, and this one sets you up to crush whatever lies ahead.

The Macros

496
Calories

32g
Protein

13g
Fat

64g
Carbs

Ideal for: Any Day
Makes 6 Servings

+ YOU'LL NEED

2 tsp grapeseed oil

2 cups small leeks, rinsed and diced

1 tbsp fresh thyme, chopped

3 cloves garlic, minced

10 oz small raw shrimp, tails off

4½ cups nonfat milk

1½ cups instant polenta

¼ tsp salt

1 cup cheddar cheese, shredded

⅓ cup Parmesan cheese, grated

2 tsp sriracha

4 eggs, beaten

Nonstick, nonfat cooking spray

+ TO MAKE IT

1 Heat a large nonstick pan over medium-high heat. Add oil, leeks, thyme, and garlic and sauté for 2 minutes, until browned.

2 Add shrimp and continue to cook for 1 minute.

3 In a large pot, bring milk to a simmer; reduce to low heat.

4 Stir in polenta and salt. Simmer for 5 minutes, stirring well throughout.

5 Remove from heat and add cheeses.

6 Place polenta mixture in a large mixing bowl and let stand for 15 minutes, stirring occasionally.

7 Stir in sriracha and eggs. Add shrimp and leek mixture and stir well.

8 Spray a casserole dish with nonstick spray. Spread polenta mixture in dish, then cover and refrigerate overnight.

9 In the morning, preheat oven to 425°. Bake uncovered for 25 minutes, or until set.

10 Finish under a high broiler for 1–2 minutes, or until slightly browned.

Muesli
with Fresh Berries
Fruity and filling, it's the perfect recovery.

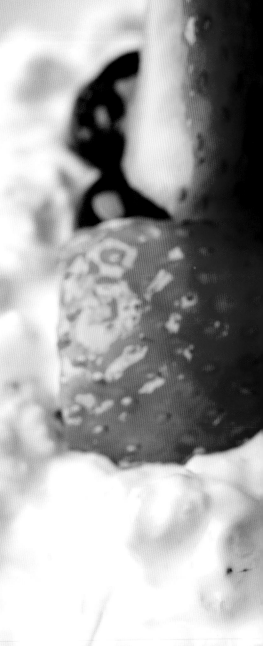

MUESLI IS GERMAN FOR "MUSH"—but please don't hold that against it! A dish made of rolled oats, nuts, and fruit, it dates back to the early 20th century, when Swiss physician and pioneer nutritionist Maximilian Bircher-Benner was looking for a way to get his patients to eat more fruit, which he considered essential to their recovery.

It's a fitting origin story, because he was right: Fruit isn't just nutrient-dense; it also contains natural sugars that can play a big role in your recovery from tough training sessions. In this recipe, you get blueberries, blackberries, strawberries, and raisins over rolled oats and nonfat Greek yogurt. The oats add cholesterol-fighting soluble fiber, and the yogurt contains healthy bacteria that can improve digestion. The calcium in yogurt also signals your body to stop producing the stress hormone cortisol—which can cause the body to store fat around your waist.

The whole mixture is sweetened with just a touch of honey (look for organic or raw when you go shopping), orange juice, whipped cream, and a dash of brown sugar. Yes, you could have just oatmeal or plain yogurt with fruit instead, but the extra steps here add only a few more carbs and make for a truly irresistible breakfast.

Ideal for: A Post-workout Meal
Makes 4 Servings

+ YOU'LL NEED

2 cups quick oats

1½ cups nonfat vanilla Greek yogurt

1 cup orange juice

2 tbsp organic or raw honey

1 tsp lemon juice

½ cup raisins

1 tbsp stevia

1 green apple, shredded
(you can use a cheese grater)

1 cup whipped cream

½ cup strawberries, quartered

¼ cup blackberries

¼ cup blueberries

+ TO MAKE IT

1 In a large bowl, mix all ingredients except whipped cream and berries. Set mixture in the fridge for 30 minutes.

2 Remove mixture and fold in whipped cream.

3 Portion muesli into bowls, top with berries, and serve.

The Macros

478
Calories

17g
Protein

12g
Fat

79g
Carbs

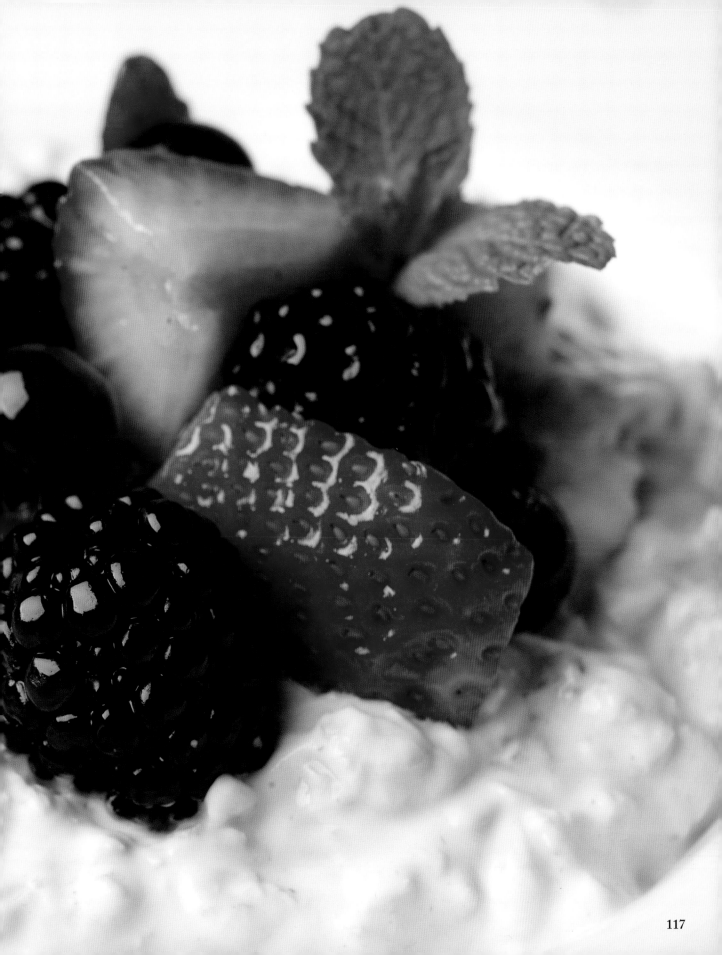

Turkey Sausage, Tomato & Spinach Frittata

Because the breakfast of champions doesn't come in a box.

BABY SPINACH AND EGGS TOGETHER—now you've got a breakfast both Popeye and Rocky Balboa would approve of! Add turkey sausage and you've got even more lean protein to round out this frittata and turn it into a perfectly balanced meal: high in protein, fiber, and healthy fats, and relatively low in carbohydrates.

I might also add that this dish is almost completely idiot-proof. It will also taste fresh for up to three days after it's baked, so you've got the green light to make extra for later in the week, when you might be short on time.

Ideal for: Any Day
Makes 2 Servings

+ YOU'LL NEED

Nonstick, nonfat cooking spray

½ **cup** turkey sausage, cooked and diced

½ **cup** onions, diced

¾ **cup** Swiss cheese, shredded

1 **cup** baby spinach leaves

1 **cup** nonfat cottage cheese

½ **cup** tomatoes, diced

½ **cup** nonfat evaporated milk

¼ **cup** reduced-fat cheddar cheese

2 whole eggs

2 egg whites

1 **tsp** baking powder

+ TO MAKE IT

1 Preheat oven to 350°.

2 Coat a large nonstick sauté pan with cooking spray and place over medium-high heat.

3 Add sausage and onions and sauté for 3 minutes, until onions are translucent. Set mixture aside.

4 Coat a 9-inch pie pan or iron skillet with cooking spray, then sprinkle ¼ cup Swiss cheese into the pan.

5 In a mixing bowl, whisk together the remaining ½ cup Swiss cheese with spinach, cottage cheese, tomatoes, evaporated milk, cheddar cheese, eggs, egg whites, and baking powder.

6 Pour egg mixture over sausage mixture, then place the pan in the oven.

7 Bake at 350° for 45 minutes, or until a knife inserted into the middle of the frittata comes out clean.

The Macros

487
Calories

47g
Protein

22g
Fat

27g
Carbs

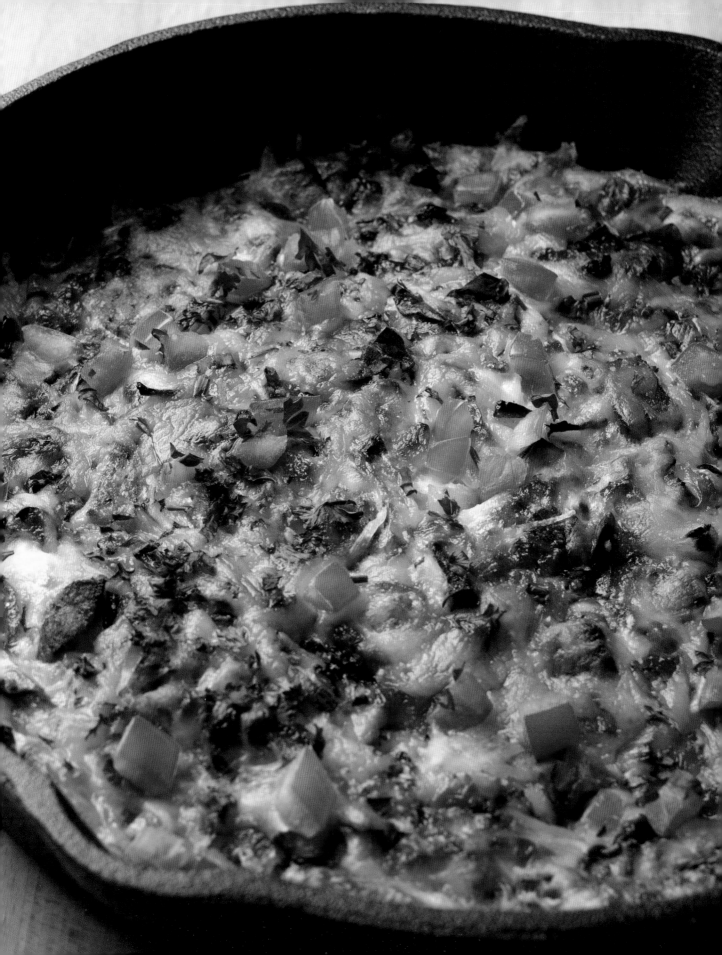

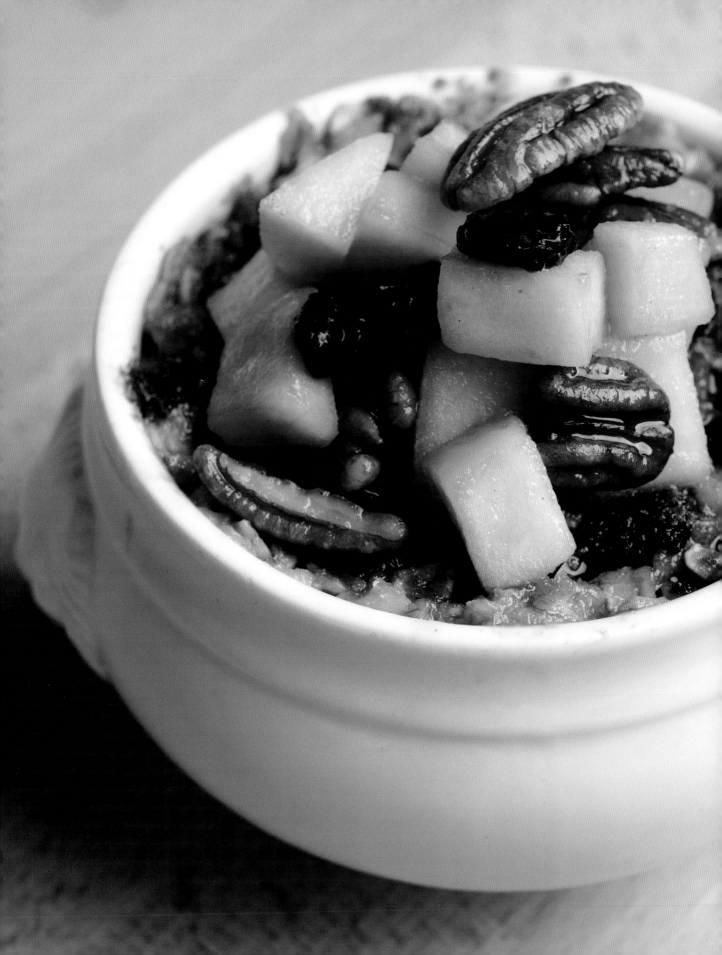

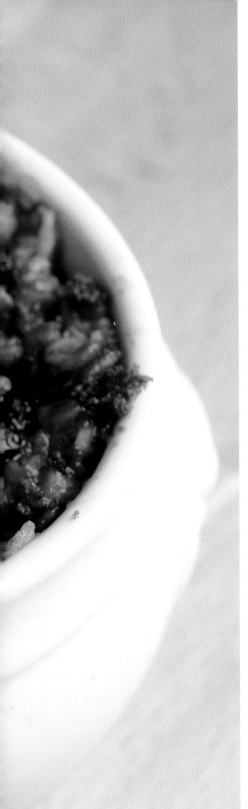

Oatmeal Brûlée
with Spiced Pear & Pecans
A sweet fiber fix.

FIBER DOES MORE THAN HELP KEEP YOU REGULAR. Hitting or exceeding your recommended daily allowance of fiber (about 30 grams, according to the USDA) can lower both your cholesterol and your risk of heart disease. Without getting too deep into the science of it, your body uses cholesterol to create bile acid, and fiber prevents that bile from being absorbed during digestion. When this happens, your body immediately tries to make more bile acid, and uses the cholesterol already in your bloodstream to do it. This, in turn, lowers total cholesterol levels.

In this recipe, the oats provide most of the fiber, but the pears also contribute. The skim milk adds protein, and the caramelized brûlée topping will make you forget you're eating anything remotely healthy.

Ideal for: A Post-workout Meal
Makes 8 Servings

The Macros

342 Calories

13g Protein

8g Fat

56g Carbs

+ YOU'LL NEED

For the Oatmeal:

8 cups nonfat milk

2 cups rolled oats

1 stick cinnamon

1 dash salt

½ cup sugar-free maple syrup

1 cup raisins (optional)

½ cup brown sugar

For the Pear & Pecan Compote:

1 tbsp butter

1 cup pears, peeled and diced

½ cup pecan halves

¼ cup sugar-free maple syrup

1 tsp lemon juice

+ TO MAKE IT

Oatmeal:

1 In a large saucepan, bring milk to a boil over medium heat. Add oats, cinnamon stick, and salt.

2 Reduce heat to a simmer, slowly stirring for 3 minutes until thick and creamy.

3 Remove from heat. Discard cinnamon stick.

4 Stir in ½ cup syrup and raisins (if desired).

Compote:

Warm butter in a sauté pan and add pears. Cook for 1 minute. Add pecans, ¼ cup syrup, and lemon juice. Bring to a simmer, then allow to cool.

To Finish:

1 Portion hot oatmeal into ovenproof bowls. Sprinkle each with brown sugar.

2 Broil in the oven for 4–6 minutes, or until brown sugar is caramelized.

3 Top with spoonful of compote.

Turkey Bacon Quesadilla
with Eggs & Avocado Salsa
The Mexican classic, made better.

THE QUESADILLA MOST PEOPLE ARE FAMILIAR WITH looks something like this: a white-flour tortilla melted shut with cheese and chicken, cut into pieces, and draped with guacamole and sour cream. Excuse me if I find this more than a bit boring. There are so many ways to get creative with quesadillas and to create healthier, more nutritionally dense variations.

We're going to cook up a savory breakfast quesadilla using whole-wheat tortillas, turkey bacon, and scrambled eggs. We'll ditch the sour cream and guac, and mix the avocado right into our fresh black bean and tomato salsa for a tangy topping that'll ensure you'll never look at quesadillas the same way again.

Ideal for: Any Day
Makes 4 Servings

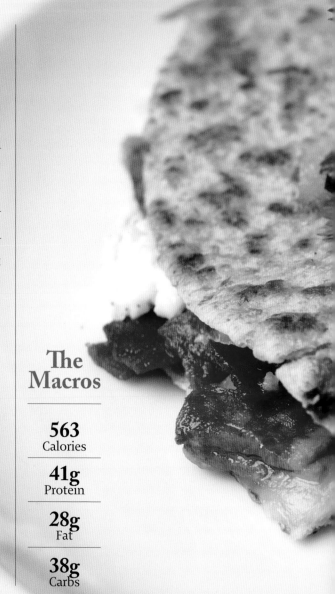

+ YOU'LL NEED

For the Avocado Salsa:
¼ **cup** black beans, rinsed

¼ **cup** tomatoes, diced

1 avocado, diced

¼ **cup** red onion, diced

¼ bunch cilantro, chopped

1 tbsp sherry vinegar

Juice of ½ lime

Salt and pepper

For the Quesadillas:
½ **cup** nonfat cottage cheese

4 12-inch whole-wheat tortillas

1 cup low-fat Jack cheese, shredded

¾ **cup** turkey bacon, cooked and chopped

Nonstick, nonfat cooking spray

For the Eggs:
1 tbsp grapeseed oil

6 whole eggs

6 egg whites

+ TO MAKE IT

Avocado Salsa:
Combine all salsa ingredients in a mixing bowl and gently toss together.

Quesadillas:
1 Spread cottage cheese on tortillas evenly, then top with Jack cheese and chopped turkey bacon.

2 Spray a nonstick pan with cooking spray; fold a tortilla in half and cook it over medium heat until cheese is melted. Repeat for all tortillas.

Eggs:
1 Heat a nonstick pan over medium heat and add 1 tbsp grapeseed oil.

2 In a mixing bowl, whisk together whole eggs and egg whites; pour eggs into pan and scramble until cooked through. Season with salt and pepper.

To Finish:
Cut each quesadilla into four pieces and arrange on the plate next to scrambled eggs. Top quesadilla with salsa.

The Macros

563
Calories

41g
Protein

28g
Fat

38g
Carbs

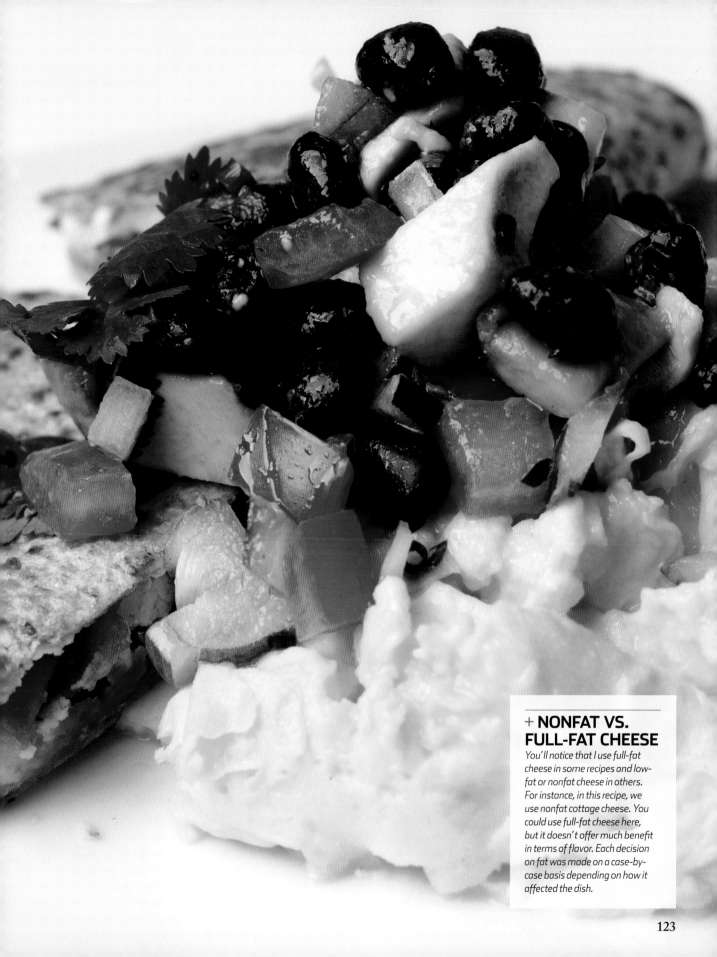

+ NONFAT VS. FULL-FAT CHEESE

You'll notice that I use full-fat cheese in some recipes and low-fat or nonfat cheese in others. For instance, in this recipe, we use nonfat cottage cheese. You could use full-fat cheese here, but it doesn't offer much benefit in terms of flavor. Each decision on fat was made on a case-by-case basis depending on how it affected the dish.

Maple Yogurt Parfait

Another perfect way to wrap up your morning workout.

AFTER A HARD TRAINING SESSION is the one time your body can actually make use of fast-digesting carbs rather than store them as fat. Hence the popularity of sports drinks like Gatorade among hard-training athletes.

Of course, there are a lot of healthier—not to mention more interesting—ways to get your post-workout carbs. Consider this Maple Yogurt Parfait as Exhibit A. Honey, maple syrup, orange juice, raisins, and a hint of brown sugar provide the fast-digesting carbs that will replenish your glycogen stores; the oats deliver sustained energy; and the Greek yogurt, walnuts, and almonds give you protein. It's sweet and decadent, yet the perfect way to refuel your body.

Ideal for: A Post-workout Meal
Makes 4 Servings

+ YOU'LL NEED

1 qt nonfat vanilla Greek yogurt

3 tbsp organic maple syrup

2 cups rolled oats

⅓ cup flaxseed meal

¼ cup walnuts, chopped

¼ cup slivered almonds

1 tsp ground cinnamon

⅓ cup orange juice

⅓ cup plus 1 tbsp honey

¼ cup brown sugar

1 tsp vanilla extract

Nonstick, nonfat cooking spray

⅓ cup golden raisins

2 tsp grapeseed oil

2 green apples, peeled and diced

+ TO MAKE IT

Yogurt:

Mix yogurt and maple syrup together in a mixing bowl. Chill in the fridge until you're ready to build the parfaits.

Granola:

1 Preheat oven to 300°.

2 Combine oats, flaxseed meal, walnuts, almonds, and cinnamon in a separate mixing bowl and set aside.

3 In a saucepan, combine OJ, ⅓ cup honey, and brown sugar on medium heat until sugar dissolves. Add vanilla and remove from heat.

4 Pour honey mixture over oat mixture. Stir together well. Coat a cookie sheet with cooking spray, then spread the mixture onto the cookie sheet.

5 Bake at 300° for 10 minutes, stir, then bake an additional 10–12 minutes, until golden brown.

6 Scrape granola into a mixing bowl and fold in raisins.

7 Allow to cool. (Store unused portion in an airtight container.)

Apples:

1 Heat grapeseed oil in a saucepan and add diced apples.

2 Sauté until tender, then add 1 tbsp honey. Coat the apples, then remove from heat and allow to cool.

To Finish:

1 Place 1 tbsp diced apple in the bottom of the glass, top with ¼ cup yogurt, then ¼ cup granola.

2 Repeat this layer one more time, then top with remaining apple. Repeat to fill all glasses, and serve.

The Macros

501
Calories

22g
Protein

10g
Fat

82g
Carbs

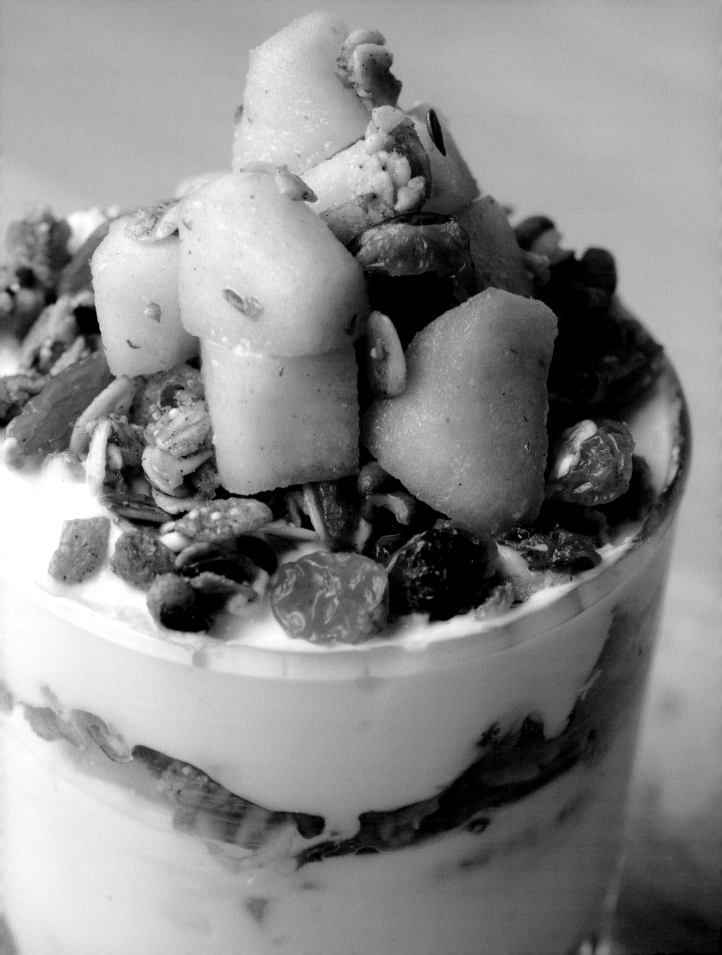

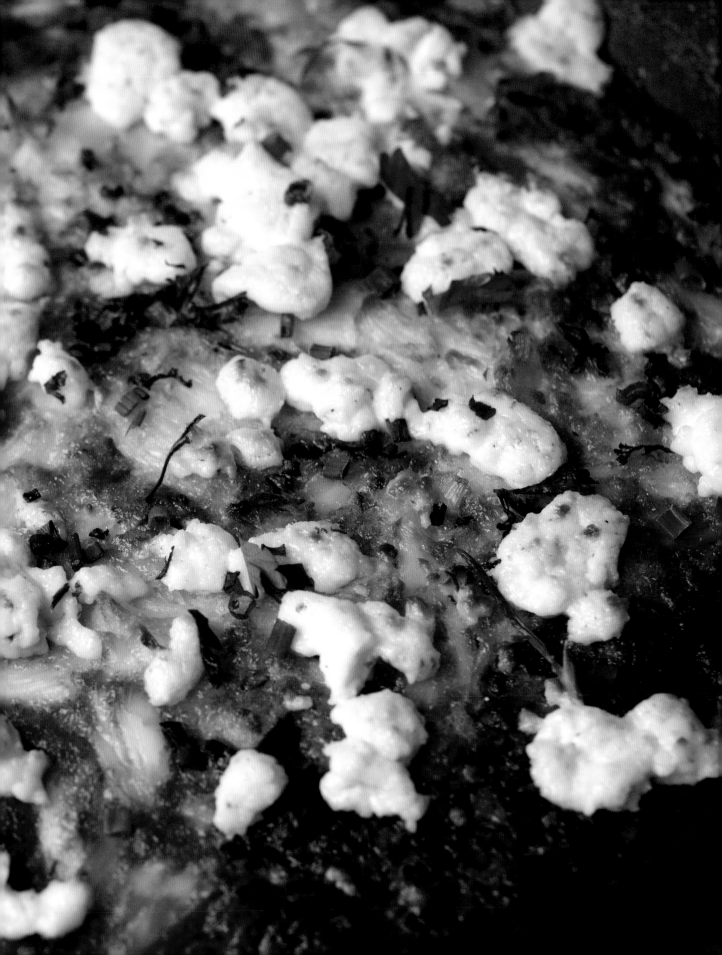

Spinach & Crab Soufflé

A meat, egg, and cheese combo that won't slow you down for the rest of the day.

BACON, EGG, AND CHEESE? Please. This Spinach & Crab Soufflé is a huge step up from the old standard, starting with the first ingredient: spinach.

I explained in the chapter on nutrition how fiber-loaded vegetables aren't just a digestion aid but also the most micronutrient-dense foods you can eat. And spinach is in a class all its own. One cup of raw spinach comes in at only 7 calories, but delivers a massive payload of vital nutrients like vitamins K and A, calcium, folate, and iron, to name just a few. It's been shown to keep blood pressure low and bones dense, and possibly even promote healthy hair and skin.

As for the whole eggs used in this recipe—there's nothing inherently unhealthy about eggs. The fat they provide serves an essential function in a healthy diet: The body uses it to produce testosterone and growth hormone. Egg yolks also contain choline, a micronutrient proven to be vital for healthy brain function.

The rich taste of the crabmeat makes this dish so satisfying, you won't miss the bacon. I'm not going to demonize bacon, since I've already explained that fats—including saturated fats—serve an important role in any diet. But having said that, it's so incredibly easy to over-eat bacon and get way more saturated fat than you need. So whenever possible, it's a good idea to replace bacon with a leaner protein source, as I've done in this recipe. Crab's protein-to-fat ratio is about 18:1. Bacon, with only slight variations depending on how it's prepared, usually has a ratio of about 1:1, making it an all-too-easy way to spend a lot of your day's calories.

The Macros

430
Calories

40g
Protein

27g
Fat

8g
Carbs

Ideal for: Any Day
Makes 2 Servings

+ YOU'LL NEED

1 tbsp grapeseed oil

½ cup onion, diced small

1 cup canned jumbo lump crabmeat

½ cup low-fat milk

1 dash ground nutmeg

1 cup spinach, chopped

8 eggs, beaten

Salt and pepper

1 tsp fresh parsley, chopped

1 tsp fresh tarragon, chopped

1 tsp fresh chives, chopped

½ cup Boursin cheese

+ TO MAKE IT

1 Preheat oven to 425°.

2 In a large, ovenproof skillet, heat oil over medium heat.

3 Sauté onion until slightly brown, about 3 minutes.

4 Add the crabmeat, milk, and nutmeg. Allow ingredients to come to a slight simmer, then add spinach. Stir until mixture starts to thicken, about 2 minutes.

5 Pour beaten eggs into skillet. Season with salt and pepper and stir until eggs are about halfway cooked.

6 Sprinkle in herbs and crumble Boursin cheese on top.

7 Place skillet in oven and cook until soufflé is set and has a light, golden color, about 12–14 minutes, then serve.

Smoked Salmon, Asparagus & Poached Eggs

The ultimate get-lean breakfast.

WHETHER YOU'RE TRYING TO LOSE FAT, add muscle, or both, salmon is one of the best types of fish you can add to your diet. The omega-3 fats in salmon don't just keep your heart healthy; they also encourage your body to burn stored fat for energy. So, yes, we're having fish for breakfast. Trust me on this one.

Salmon has a distinctive flavor. The only thing I like more than fresh salmon is smoked salmon, which adds even more delicious layers. When we pair it with blanched asparagus, poached eggs, frisée lettuce, and watercress, we get a high-protein, high-fiber, low-carb meal that will satisfy you *and* fuel your fitness goals.

When you're shopping, look for wild smoked salmon. Wild salmon contains more calcium, iron, zinc, and potassium than its farm-raised counterpart, and also has fewer calories, owing to the fact it has just a third of the saturated fat of the farm-raised variety.

Ideal for: Any Day
Makes 4 Servings

+ YOU'LL NEED

16 asparagus spears

½ cup white vinegar

8 organic eggs

12 slices wild smoked salmon

2 tbsp grapeseed oil

Juice of **½** lemon

Salt and pepper

1 bunch frisée lettuce

1 bunch watercress

¼ cup red onion, thinly julienned

1 tbsp capers

1 tbsp fresh chives, chopped

+ TO MAKE IT

1 Blanch asparagus by boiling in water for no more than 3 minutes (the spears should turn bright green), then placing in ice water for about a minute.

2 In a pot, bring 2 qts water almost to a boil; add vinegar.

3 Crack one egg into a small cup. Hold the cup near the surface of the water. Gently drop the egg into the hot water. Repeat this process with each egg.

4 With a spoon, gently nudge egg whites closer to yolks; this, along with the vinegar, will help whites hold together. Cook eggs for about 4 minutes.

5 Remove pot from heat and allow eggs to sit in water until ready to plate.

6 Arrange 3 pieces of salmon in a flat circle on each plate.

7 Place asparagus in a mixing bowl and toss with grapeseed oil, lemon juice, salt, and pepper.

8 Arrange 4 asparagus spears in the middle of each plate.

9 Place frisée, watercress, red onion, and capers in the same mixing bowl with the leftover lemon juice and grapeseed oil. Add salt and pepper and toss.

10 Arrange a small bed of salad in the middle of each plate, and top each salad with 2 poached eggs. Garnish eggs with chopped chives.

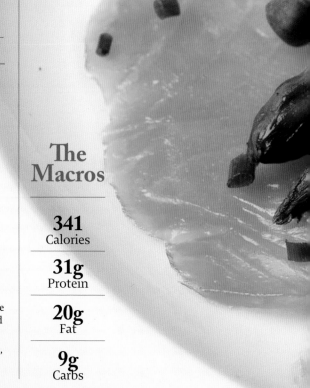

The Macros

341
Calories

31g
Protein

20g
Fat

9g
Carbs

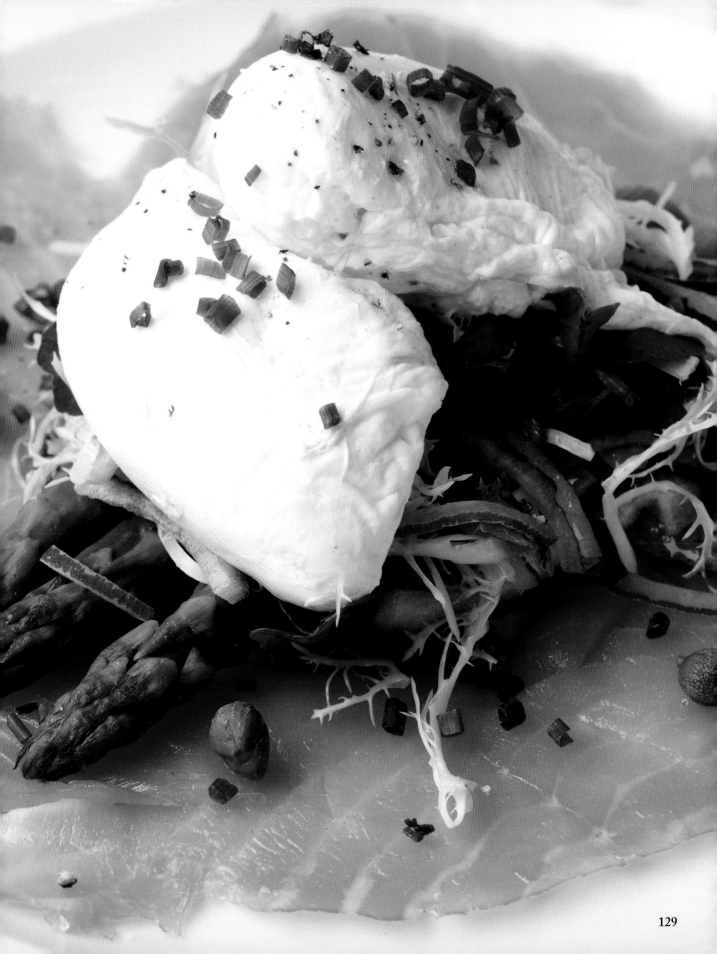

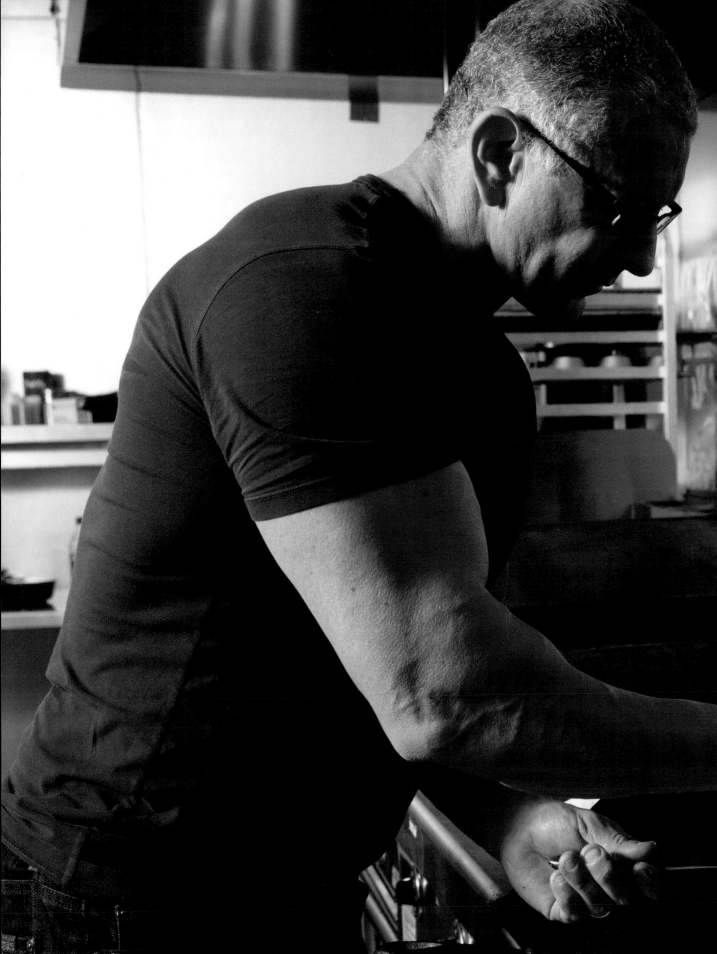

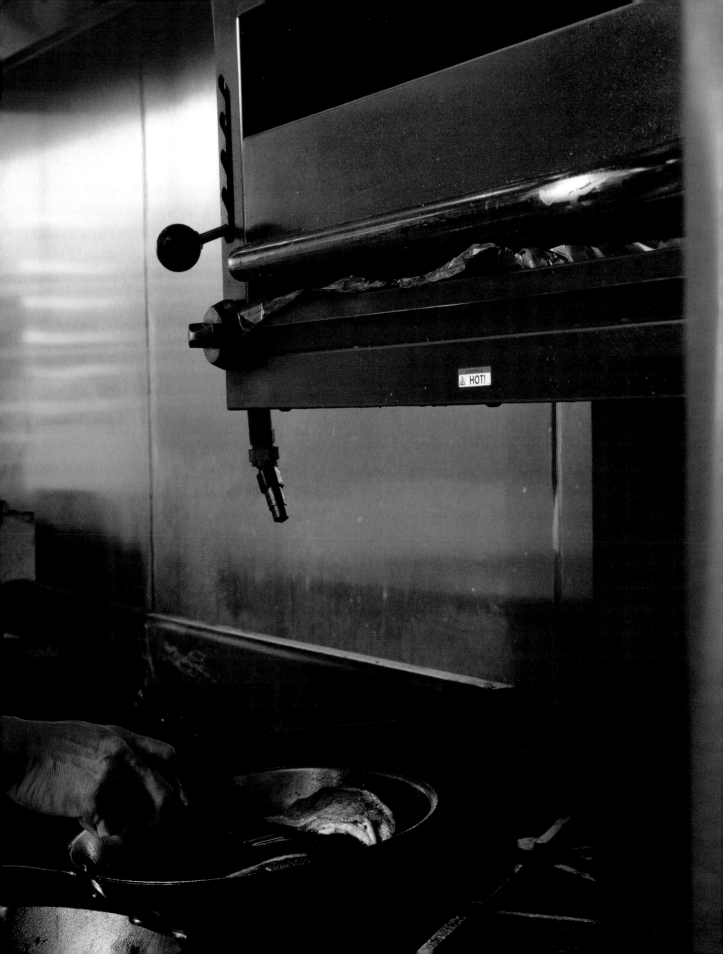

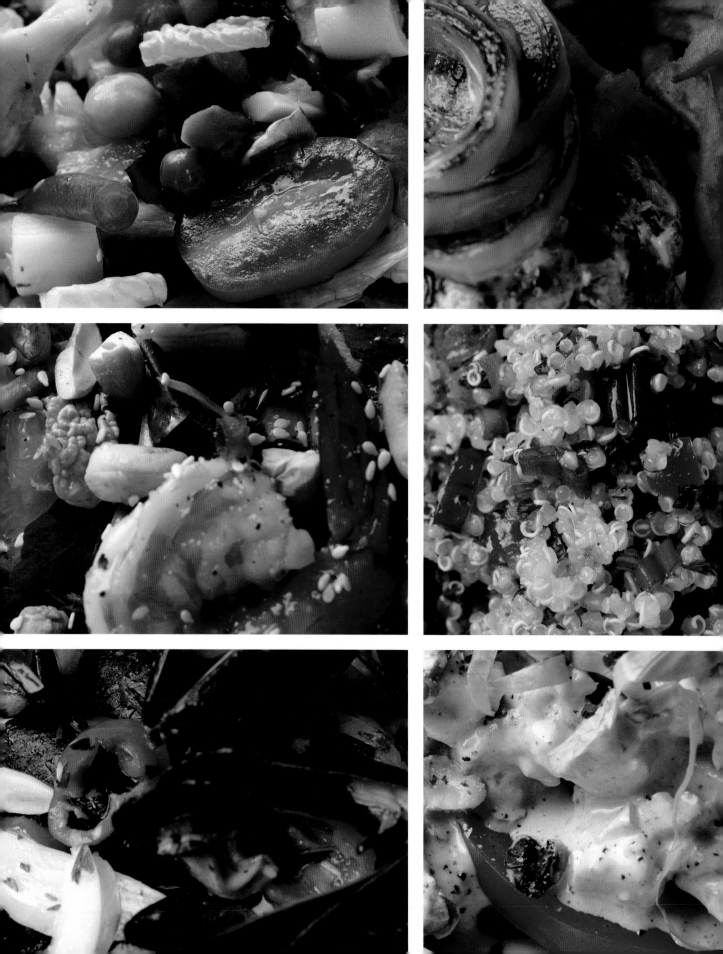

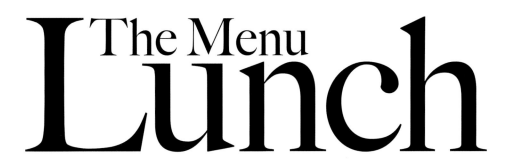

The Menu
Lunch

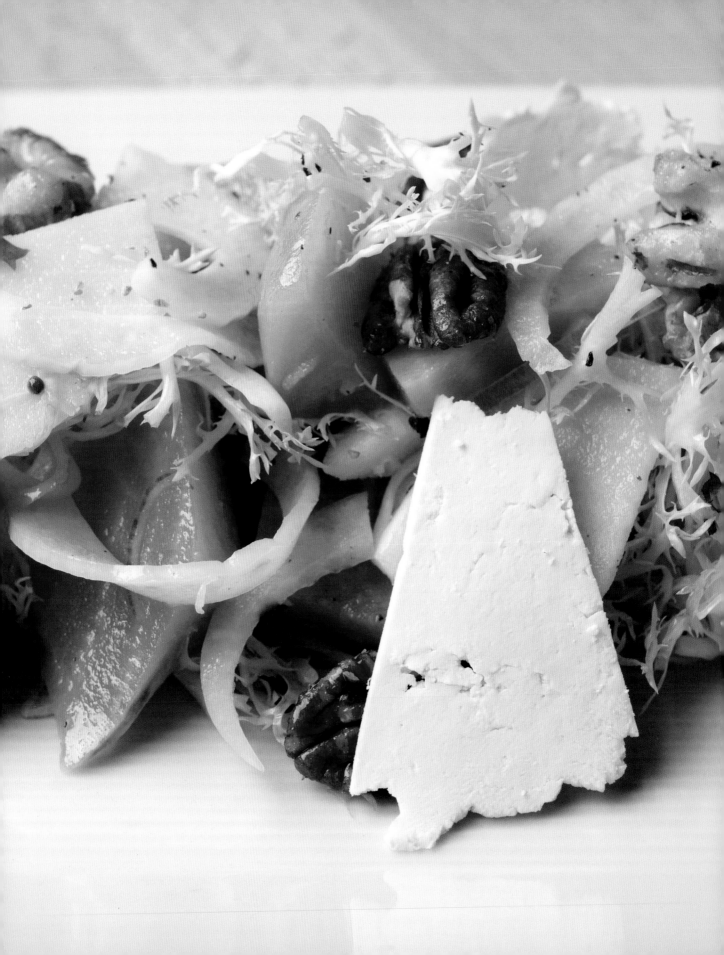

Roasted Beet Salad

A nutrient-dense option for the whole family.

YOUR MOTHER MAY NOT HAVE KNOWN the science behind it when she scolded you into eating your vegetables, but this *is* one of the most important things you can do to get fit. In light of recent studies, her advice makes more sense now than ever.

And this salad has one of the most potent vegetables of all. Research has shown that beets—and particularly beet juice—can boost athletic performance and endurance. More benefits of this dish: The walnuts and pecans provide healthy fats and protein, and the saturated fat in the cheese will keep you feeling satisfied for longer.

The Macros

362
Calories

11g
Protein

23g
Fat

36g
Carbs

Ideal for: Any Day
Makes 4 Servings

+ YOU'LL NEED

For the Beets:
- 1 cup salt
- 12 sprigs thyme
- 2 lbs yellow beets, washed

For the Nuts:
- ½ cup walnut halves
- ½ cup pecan halves
- 2 tbsp honey
- ½ tsp salt
- 1 tbsp water

For the Salad:
- 2 shallots, thinly julienned
- 4 oz fennel, thinly julienned
- 1 green apple, peeled and sliced
- Salt and pepper
- 4 heads frisée lettuce, rinsed and patted dry
- 20 shavings ricotta salata
- Fat-free dressing of your choice

+ TO MAKE IT

Beets:
1 Preheat oven to 350°.

2 Spread salt on a sheet pan and evenly place thyme and beets on top of the salt bed. Cover with foil and place in the oven for 60–90 minutes, until tender. To check doneness, poke beets with a toothpick. Peel beets (it's easier to do when they're warm) and set them aside. Don't turn oven off.

Nuts:
1 Toss nuts in a bowl with honey, water, and salt.

2 Spread nuts on a sheet pan and place in oven for 5-6 minutes, until lightly toasted.

Salad:
1 Slice beets into small wedges. Put beet wedges, julienned shallots, fennel, and sliced apple in a large bowl. Toss and season with salt and pepper.

2 Add frisée and toss lightly.

To Finish:
Portion onto plates and serve topped with toasted nuts, shaved cheese, and dressing.

Chopped Farm Salad

Deep country flavors in just a few minutes.

THE EVER-INCREASING POPULARITY of the salad bag has to be one of the saddest supermarket trends I've witnessed in my lifetime. A fresh, creative, and delicious salad takes about 5–10 minutes. Why settle for a bland, factory-assembled salad if you don't have to?

My Chopped Farm Salad with tomato Provençal dressing is a perfect balance of bitter (garlic, vinegar) and sweet (honey) flavors as well as crisp (romaine, radicchio, asparagus, green beans, cucumber) and creamy (chickpeas, artichokes) textures. When that combination hits your taste buds, you'll be glad you didn't take the lazy way out with the salad bag.

Ideal for: Any Day
Makes 8 Servings

+ YOU'LL NEED

For the Dressing:

1 red pepper, cleaned of seeds

3 oz tomato juice

1 tbsp dried oregano

1 tbsp chopped garlic

6 oz white vinegar

½ cup blended oil (olive and vegetable)

¼ cup honey

1 shallot, roughly cut

Salt and pepper

For the Salad:

3 heads romaine lettuce, chopped

½ head radicchio lettuce, chopped

½ cup asparagus, blanched and cut on a bias

½ cup artichokes, quartered

½ cup green beans, blanched, cut in 1-inch pieces

½ cup green peas

½ cup cucumber, diced

½ cup grape tomatoes, halved

½ cup hearts of palm, sliced thick

½ cup chickpeas

Salt and pepper

+ TO MAKE IT

Dressing:
Mix all dressing ingredients well in a blender, slowly adding oil throughout. Season with salt and pepper.

Salad:
1 Place all salad ingredients into a large mixing bowl and toss with dressing. Season with salt and pepper.
2 Serve in one large salad bowl or portion into smaller bowls.

The Macros

159
Calories

5g
Protein

17g
Fat

28g
Carbs

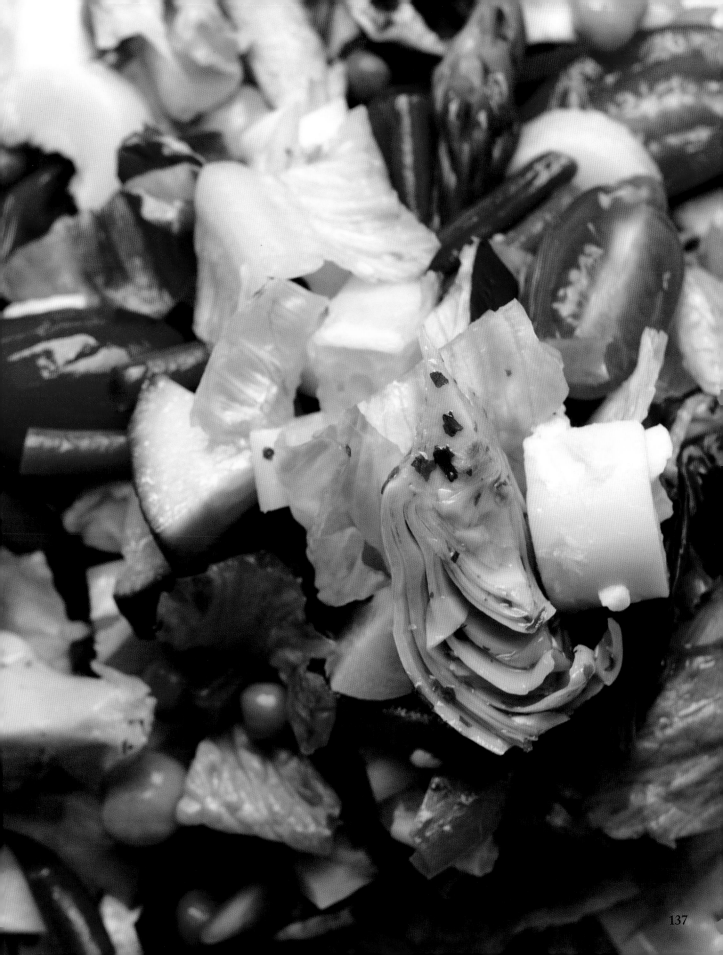

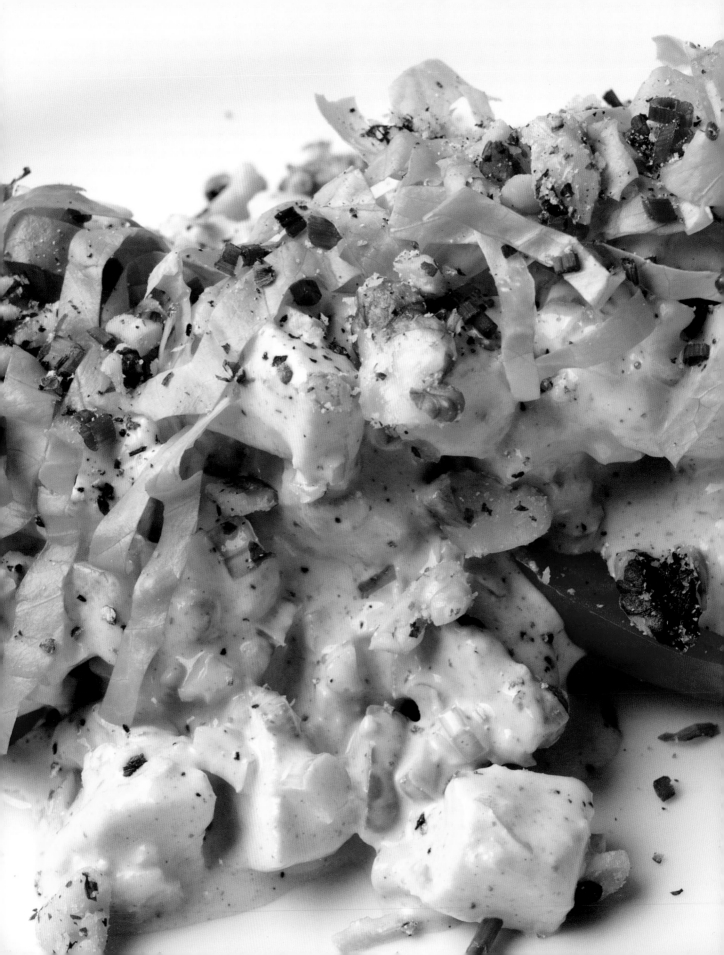

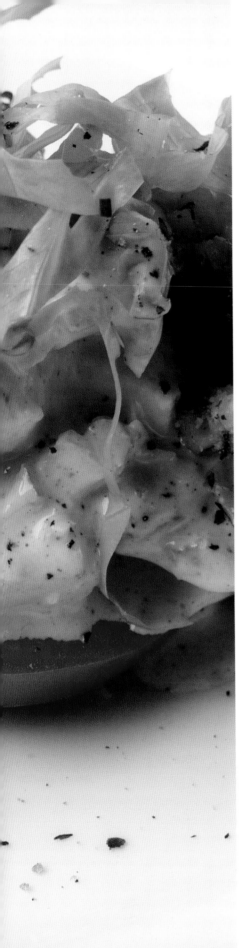

Curried Chicken Salad Lettuce Wraps
Low-carb and loving it.

YOU MIGHT BE SURPRISED HOW LITTLE you'd miss bread if you tried just one of your favorite sandwiches without it. If you've got good ingredients and interesting flavor combinations, those elements should be enough to carry a satisfying meal without any help from a huge hunk of processed carbs.

That's certainly the case with these Curried Chicken Salad Lettuce Wraps. The spiciness of the curry balances the sweetness of the mango chutney and grapes. Plus, the walnuts and celery add a satisfying snap. Served in Bibb lettuce leaves—or eaten straight up with a fork—it's a terrific low-carb lunch or late-afternoon snack that will give you energy without any crash.

The Macros

409
Calories

40g
Protein

23g
Fat

12g
Carbs

Ideal for: Any Day
Makes 4 Servings (each serving is 3 wraps)

+ YOU'LL NEED

3 cups chicken breast, cooked and diced

1 stalk celery, minced

½ cup grapes, halved

½ cup walnuts

1 tsp lemon juice

½ cup mayonnaise

1 tsp Madras curry powder

¼ tsp mango chutney

Salt and pepper

12 Bibb lettuce leaves

1 tomato, sliced

+ TO MAKE IT

1 In a mixing bowl, combine all ingredients except lettuce leaves. Mix until an even consistency is reached.

2 Place chicken salad in the middle of a large platter and arrange lettuce leaves and tomato around it to serve family-style. You can also store it in the fridge and portion chicken salad into each lettuce leaf when you're ready to eat.

Quinoa Tabbouleh

A meat-free masterpiece.

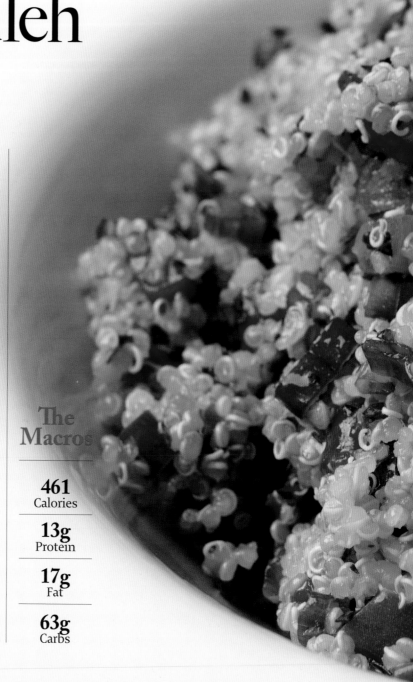

I PLACE QUINOA IN A RARE CATEGORY of supergrains that contain no gluten, induce no significant insulin spike (or subsequent energy crash), and are high in protein (8 grams per cooked cup) and fiber (5 grams per cooked cup). If every grain were like quinoa, I think more people would find it easy to go vegetarian, at least from time to time. This quinoa tabbouleh (a type of Eastern Mediterranean salad) is both filling and flavorful. It's customary to serve a tabbouleh with pita chips or lavash (an unleavened flat bread), but if you're watching carbs, it also stands well on its own.

Ideal for: Any Day
Makes 8 Servings

+ YOU'LL NEED

1 **lb** raw quinoa

1½ qts water

⅓ **cup** lemon juice

¼ **cup** extra-virgin olive oil

¼ **cup** grapeseed oil

2 **cups** tomatoes, diced small

⅓ **cup** mint, finely chopped

¾ **cup** parsley, finely chopped

1 bunch scallion, finely chopped

Salt and pepper

4 pieces lavash bread, cut in half

+ TO MAKE IT

1 Rinse quinoa with cold water in a China cap strainer and place in a pot with the water. Bring to a simmer, then turn to low heat and cover. Continue to cook for 10–12 minutes, which will yield slightly al dente quinoa.

2 Once it's cooled, place quinoa in a large bowl with all other ingredients and mix well.

3 Place in a serving bowl and serve with lavash.

The Macros

461
Calories

13g
Protein

17g
Fat

63g
Carbs

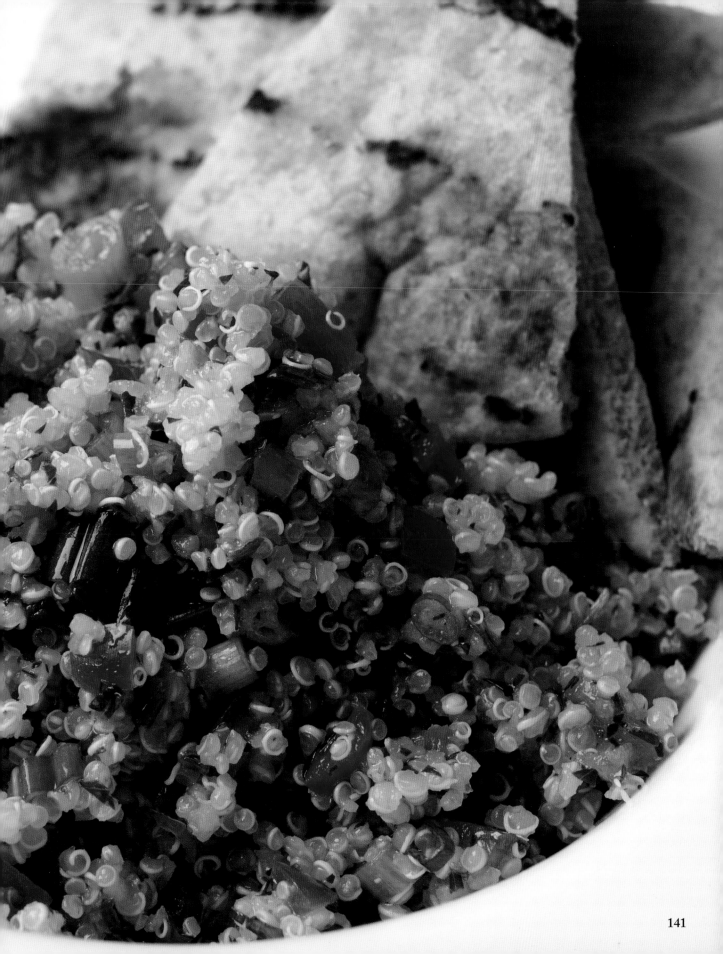

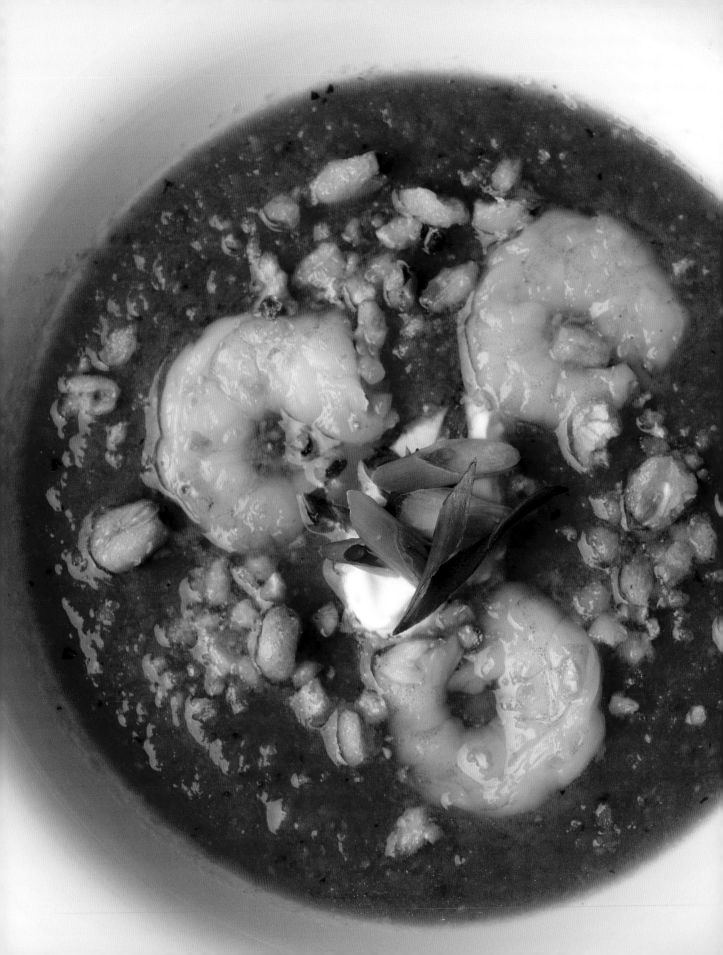

Summer Gazpacho
with Chilled Shrimp, Lime Crema & Corn Nuts
Exotic Spanish flavor—savory and refreshing.

THIS IS A PERFECT EXAMPLE OF A DISH that can combat overeating. One reason many people overeat is because their meals fail to satisfy—often because the food is devoid of distinct flavors. The key, then, is to fill your diet with as many flavorful, healthy options as possible.

Brimming with herbs and vegetables and prepared without a lot of extra fat, this shrimp gazpacho fits all the requirements of a healthy diet—and then some. The flavors are bright and tangy, and there's just enough protein to make it a well-rounded meal. To boot, it's refreshing when cold. You can make it and serve it right away, family-style, or eat it throughout the week, as it keeps well in the fridge.

The Macros

303
Calories

13g
Protein

15g
Fat

31g
Carbs

Ideal for: Any Day
(Especially when cravings attack!) *Makes 4 Servings*

+ YOU'LL NEED

For the Gazpacho:
- **10** plum tomatoes, halved
- **½** red pepper, rough cut
- **½** stalk fennel, rough cut
- **½** cucumber, rough cut
- **¼** bunch cilantro, rinsed
- **¼** bunch basil, rinsed
- **3** stalks celery
- **2** cloves garlic
- **¼** red onion, chopped
- **3 tbsp** lemon juice
- **¼ cup** grapeseed oil
- **1 dash** cumin
- **1 tsp** tabasco
- **4 tbsp** red vinegar
- **3 cups** tomato juice
- **1 tsp** Worcestershire sauce
- Salt and pepper

For the Lime Crema:
- **4 tsp** low-fat sour cream
- **½ tsp** low-fat milk
- Juice of ½ lime

For the Shrimp:
- **12** medium shrimp, cooked, tails removed
- **¼ cup** scallions, chopped
- **4 tsp** corn nuts, chopped

+ TO MAKE IT

Gazpacho:
1. With a hand blender, blend all tomatoes together.
2. Add all other gazpacho ingredients except salt and pepper, and blend until it's an even consistency. Season with salt and pepper.
3. Chill for at least 30 minutes.

Lime Crema:
In a mixing bowl, mix all ingredients together with a spoon.

To Finish:
1. Pour chilled gazpacho evenly into bowls. Spoon ¼ of lime crema into the center of each bowl.
2. Arrange 3 shrimp around lime crema and garnish with chopped scallion and corn nuts.

Prince Edward Island Mussels

Comfort food fit for royalty.

PRINCE EDWARD ISLAND MUSSELS (or PEI mussels) are known for being the best mussels you can buy. Raised in an ideal environment—the crisp, clean Canadian waters off Prince Edward Island—these mussels grow to a plump and meaty size, with shells that are free of the typical grit and sand.

It's a shame to eat a delicacy like this and skimp on the butter, so I made it a relatively rich dish (preferably to eat on a day when you train hard), with fennel, garlic, grapeseed oil, and butter, and served with a French baguette.

High in protein with a potent flavor bouquet, this is a way to let yourself indulge just a bit, but without taking in empty calories.

Ideal for: A Hard Training Day *Makes 4 Servings*

+ YOU'LL NEED

2 tbsp grapeseed oil

½ bulb fennel, thinly julienned

1 tbsp red chilies, thinly sliced

4 cloves garlic, slivered

2 lbs PEI mussels

1 cup extra-dry vermouth

1 cup red and yellow cherry tomatoes

2 tbsp smooth Dijon mustard

Juice of 1 lemon

2 tbsp salted butter

½ bunch chopped parsley

Salt and pepper

8 slices French baguette

+ TO MAKE IT

1 Place a large stockpot over medium-high heat and add grapeseed oil. Allow oil to get hot, then add fennel, chilies, garlic, and mussels.

2 Stir and allow garlic to become fragrant and light golden brown in color.

3 Deglaze mussels with vermouth.

4 Add tomatoes, mustard, lemon juice, and butter to pan. Cover and allow to steam for 3–4 minutes.

5 Once mussels have opened (discard any that don't open), add chopped parsley and season with salt and pepper.

6 Toast baguette slices under a broiler for about a minute. (Watch them closely.) Serve mussels in bowls with broth and slices of toasted baguette.

The Macros

587 Calories

36g Protein

19g Fat

53g Carbs

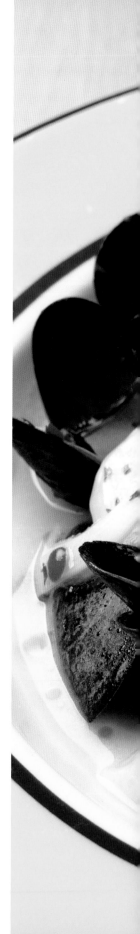

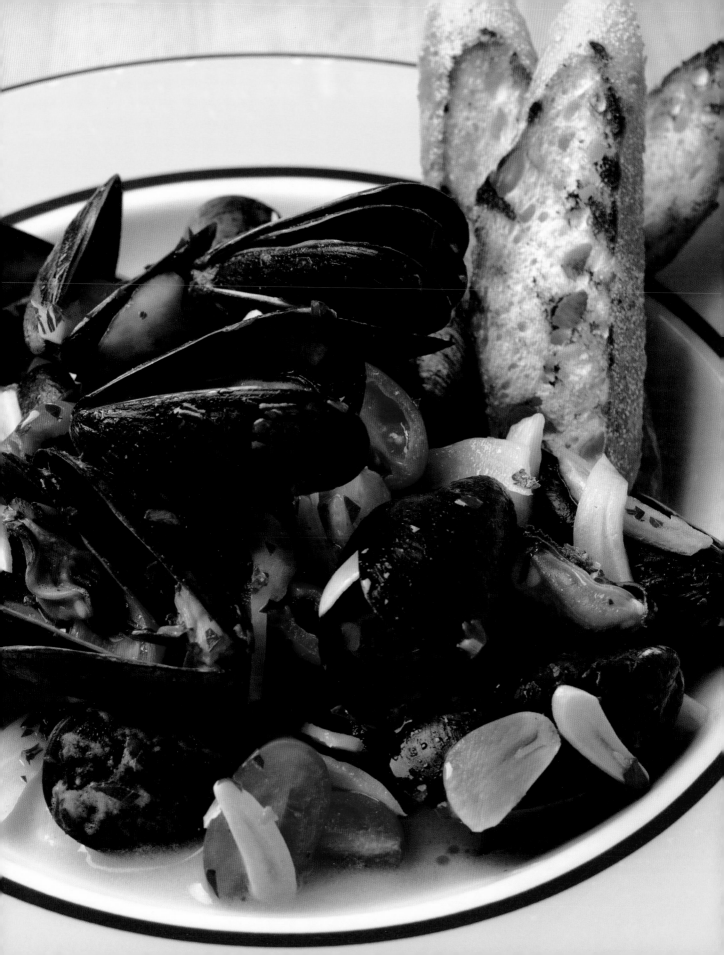

Puttanesca Tuna Burgers

Quite possibly the world's healthiest burger.

I DON'T REALLY BELIEVE there's much that can take the place of a steak. The rich taste, the fat, the juice, the way it fills you up—healthier options don't really replicate that. Burgers, though, are something of a different story. The enjoyment of eating a burger isn't necessarily tied to the kind of protein (typically ground beef) in the center of the bun. The bun itself and the toppings can often overshadow what's in the middle.

With that in mind, I've ditched the beef and instead created these Puttanesca Tuna Burgers, which are rich, flavorful, and don't pack even a fraction of the fat that comes with a typical 80:20 burger (80% meat, 20% fat, the standard at most restaurants).

Any burger can help you build muscle—this one can help get you lean, too.

Ideal for: Any Day
Makes 8 Servings

+ YOU'LL NEED

For the Patties:

3½ lbs fresh raw tuna

3 tbsp capers, minced

3 tbsp raisins, minced

1 tsp garlic, minced

3 tbsp black olives, minced

3 tbsp red onion, minced

1 tsp dried oregano

½ tsp red pepper flakes

⅓ cup parsley, chopped

3 tbsp toasted pine nuts

⅓ cup extra-virgin olive oil

Salt and pepper

Nonfat, nonstick cooking spray

For the Burgers:

8 whole-wheat hamburger rolls

8 tbsp basil pesto

8 slices red onion, grilled

1 cup roasted red peppers

+ TO MAKE IT

1 Preheat grill to 350°.

2 Dice tuna, then put it in a food processor and give it a rough mince, about 15 seconds, so it can be molded. (It should not be puréed.)

3 Remove tuna from food processor and place in a chilled mixing bowl. Mix all other patty ingredients in with it by hand. Season with salt and pepper, then portion into eight 7-oz patties.

4 Spray each side of patties with cooking spray.

5 Place patties on grill and cook 4 minutes on each side; this will yield a medium (pink) center.

6 If desired, grill rolls for 1 minute. Spread 1 tbsp pesto inside each roll. Place patties on buns, and top with onion and red peppers.

The Macros

585
Calories

68g
Protein

26g
Fat

22g
Carbs

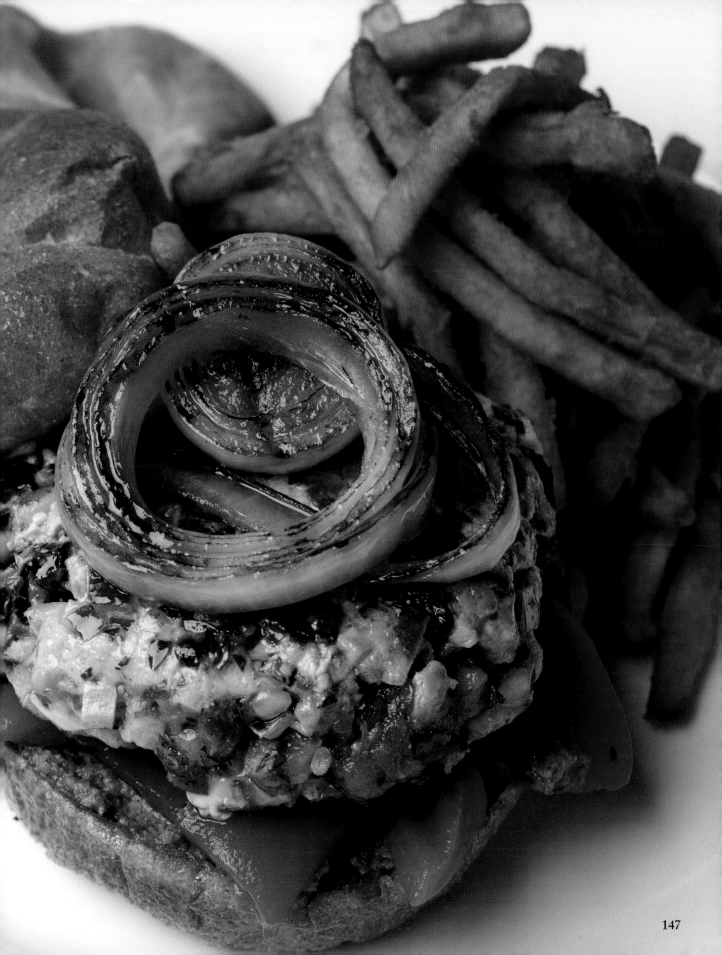

Whole-Wheat Turkey Wraps

Good to go.

IT SEEMS EVERY CHAIN RESTAURANT in the world now has some kind of wrap option. Gas stations and mini-marts, too. I know, because in my travels I've tried more wraps than I could ever possibly remember. Did they live up to my standards? Few things do!

Here, I've perfected a way to take a boring old turkey wrap and make it memorable, even if there's no fresh turkey on hand and you have to make do with deli meat.

I accomplish that with a few ingredients you probably wouldn't consider typical for a wrap: Brie cheese, orange marmalade, cranberry sauce, and white wine vinegar. These give the perfect balance of tart and sweet, and just the right amount of carbs—not the overload you might get from a sandwich.

Ideal for: Any Day
Makes 4 Servings

+ YOU'LL NEED

6 tbsp whole-grain mustard

2 tbsp light mayonnaise

3 tbsp orange marmalade

½ cup canned whole-berry cranberry sauce

1 tsp white wine vinegar

4 whole-wheat wraps

1 bunch watercress

1 lb sliced deli turkey meat

4 oz Brie cheese, cut into 8 thin pieces

Toothpicks

+ TO MAKE IT

1 In a small mixing bowl, mix together mustard and mayonnaise and set aside. In another small mixing bowl, combine orange marmalade, cranberry sauce, and vinegar, and set aside.

2 Lay whole-wheat wraps on a clean work surface and spread 2 tbsp of each sauce in center of each wrap. Divide watercress evenly among wraps, placing it on top of sauces.

3 Top watercress with 4 oz turkey and two pieces of Brie.

4 Fold sides of each wrap toward the center, then roll it up from bottom to top. Place toothpicks on each end of each wrap, then cut wraps in half.

The Macros

402 Calories	25g Protein	17g Fat	38g Carbs

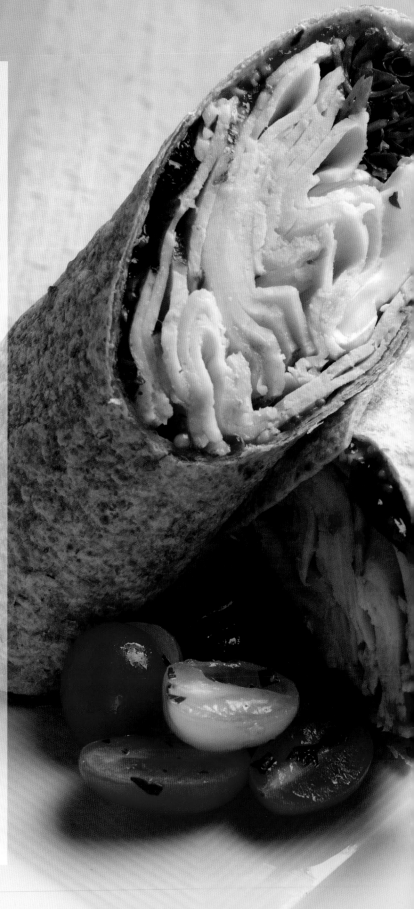

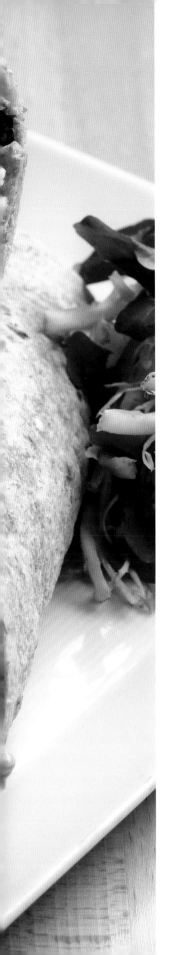

Grilled Octopus Niçoise Salad

If you're afraid of a little octopus, then you're missing out—big time.

TO MANY PEOPLE, ESPECIALLY AMERICANS, octopus is, unfortunately, an undiscovered treat. It's high in protein, low in overall calories and fat (less than 2 grams of fat in a 3-oz portion), and contains a good dose of taurine, a powerful amino acid that boosts focus (it's one of the active ingredients in energy shots like 5-hour Energy)—and may also help fight heart disease.

When it's prepared properly, octopus is a culinary delight with few rivals, because it's versatile enough to take on a wide palette of flavors. If you've got a little bit of time to make this grilled octopus salad with Niçoise olives, your whole family will be in for a treat as delicious as it is healthy.

Ideal for: Any Day
Makes 8 Servings

The Macros

566
Calories

72g
Protein

18g
Fat

27g
Carbs

+ YOU'LL NEED

For the Octopus:
1 **cup** carrots, diced large
1 **cup** onion, diced large
1 **cup** celery, diced large
1 bay leaf
1 lemon, halved
½ **cup** red wine vinegar
4 cloves garlic
¼ **cup** salt
2 gallons water
4 **lbs** Spanish octopus, uncooked
1 **cup** balsamic vinaigrette

For the Salad:
1 **qt** baby arugula
4 heads frisée lettuce
½ head radicchio lettuce, chopped
½ **cup** Niçoise olives, pitted
1 **cup** green beans, blanched and cut
1 **cup** baby Yukon Gold potatoes, quartered and cooked
½ bunch flat-leaf parsley sprigs
1 shallot, shaved
3 eggs, hard-boiled
½ **cup** grape tomatoes, halved

+ TO MAKE IT

1 Preheat grill to 350°.

2 In large pot, add carrots, onion, celery, bay leaf, lemon, vinegar, garlic, and salt to water and bring to a boil.

3 Add raw octopus, lower to a simmer, and cook for 30-45 minutes, until tender. Remove octopus and allow to cool on a sheet pan in the fridge.

4 Once octopus is chilled, remove the beak from the center of the body on the bottom side. Cut octopus into sections, removing each tentacle at its base, and place in a mixing bowl. Marinate octopus with ½ cup of the balsamic vinaigrette.

5 Place marinated octopus on grill and allow to char, occasionally brushing with leftover marinade.

6 When octopus is almost done—it will begin to char after 4–5 minutes—mix rest of salad ingredients together with remaining balsamic vinaigrette.

7 Cut some of the grilled octopus and mix it with the salad; arrange salad on a large platter.

8 Slice remainder of octopus and arrange it on top of and around salad.

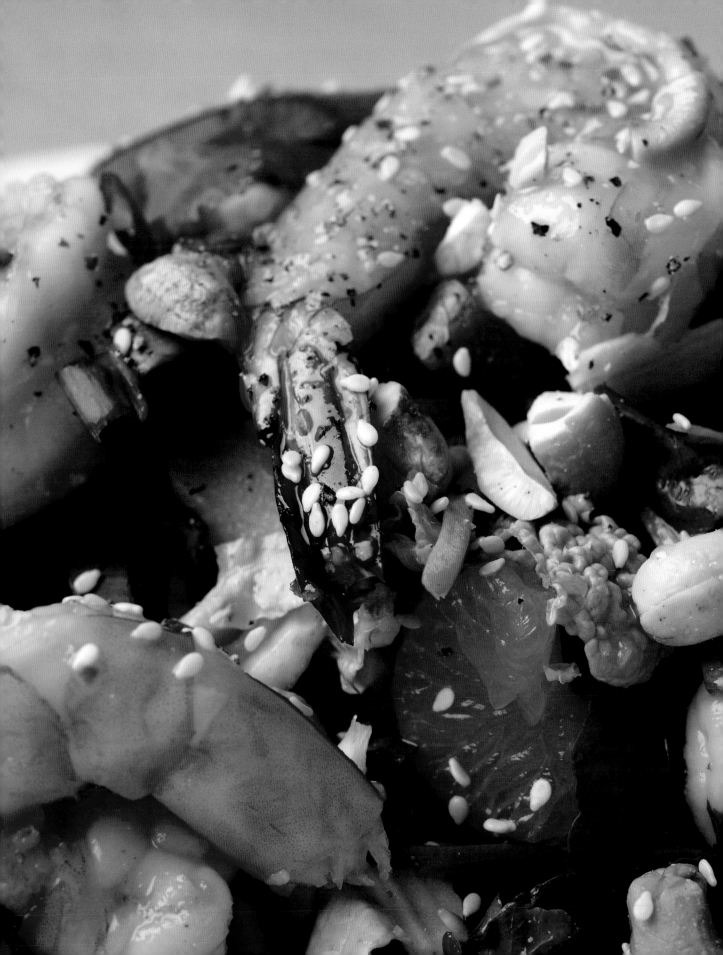

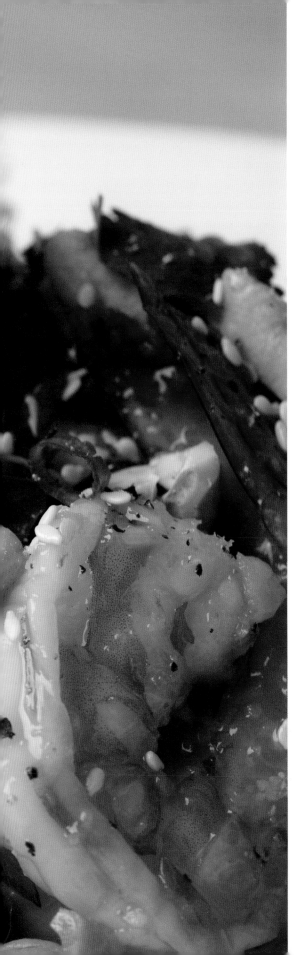

Sesame Shrimp Chopped Salad

Enchantment under the sea.

SHRIMP IS WILDLY UNDERRATED when it comes to the health benefits it offers. Though we consider most seafood to be a good source of omega-3 fatty acids, shrimp is especially high in them: A quarter-pound serving yields more than 350 mg of omega-3s. Shrimp is also one of the best whole-food sources of astaxanthin, a powerful anti-inflammatory and antioxidant.

As for sesame seeds, most people think of them as a sort of throwaway condiment, a take-it-or-leave-it topping for buns and bagels. But sesame seeds actually contain good amounts of calcium, magnesium, iron, zinc, B1, selenium (important for fertility in both men and women), and fiber.

Ideal for: Any Day

Makes 6 Servings

The Macros

222
Calories

14g
Protein

11g
Fat

19g
Carbs

+ YOU'LL NEED

- **1 cup** medium shrimp, cooked, tails removed
- **½ cup** carrots, shredded
- **½ cup** cucumber, diced small
- **1** small head napa cabbage, julienned
- **1** bunch watercress
- **½ cup** canned mandarin oranges in juice, drained
- **½ cup** canned water chestnuts
- **½** bunch cilantro sprigs
- **1 cup** celery, diced
- **1** bunch scallions, chopped
- **¾ cup** Asian sesame ginger dressing
- **½ cup** roasted cashews, chopped
- **1 tbsp** toasted sesame seeds

+ TO MAKE IT

1. Place all ingredients except cashews and sesame seeds in a large mixing bowl, and toss.
2. Place salad in a large serving bowl or on a platter. Sprinkle with cashews and sesame seeds and serve.

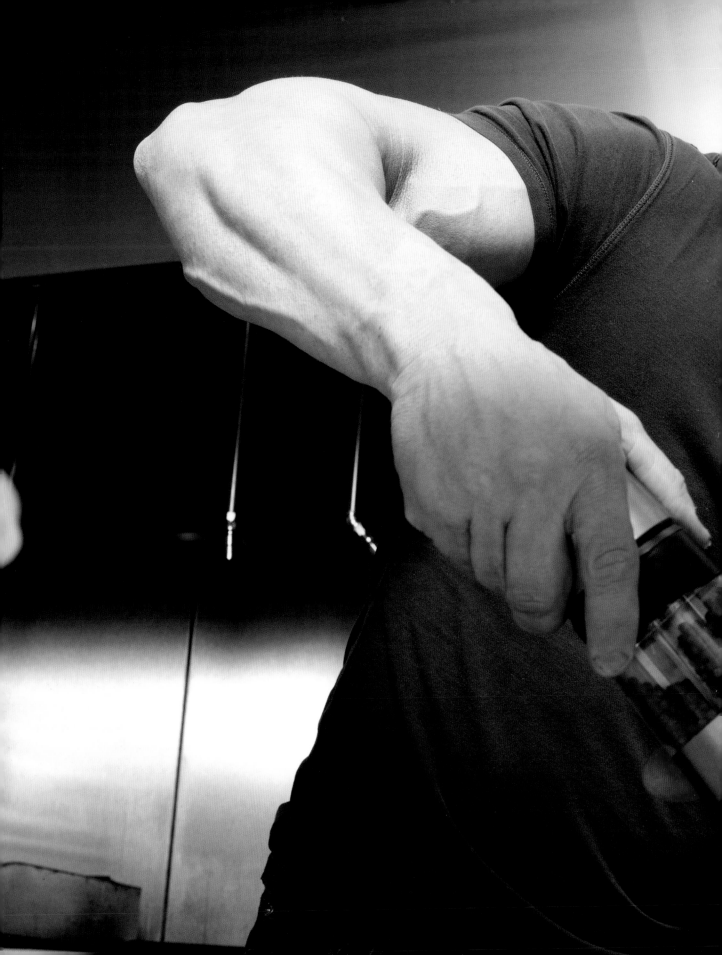

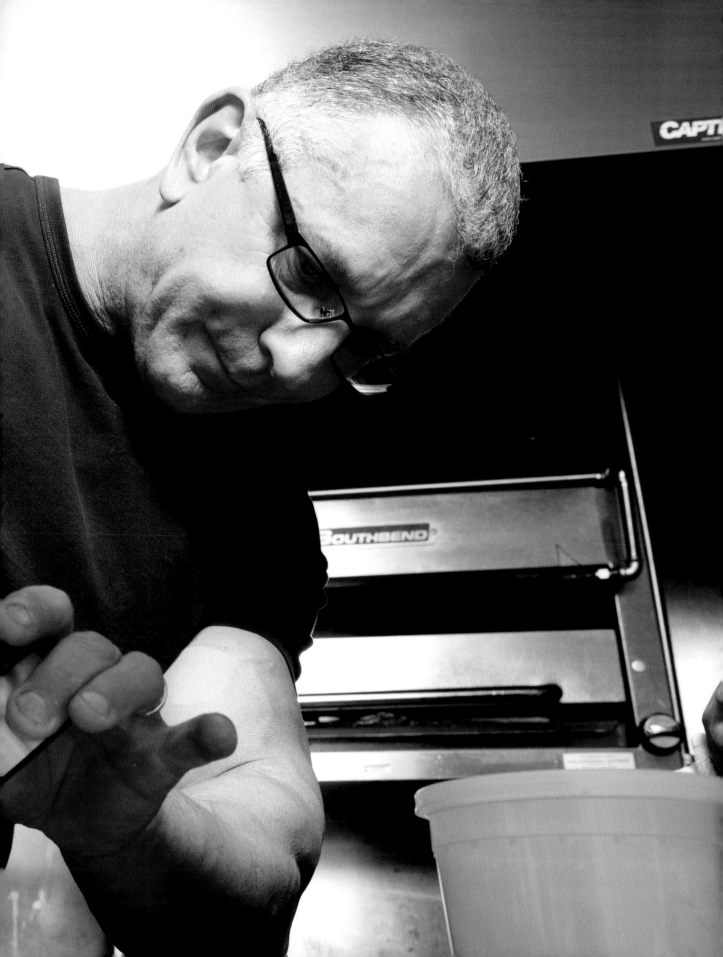

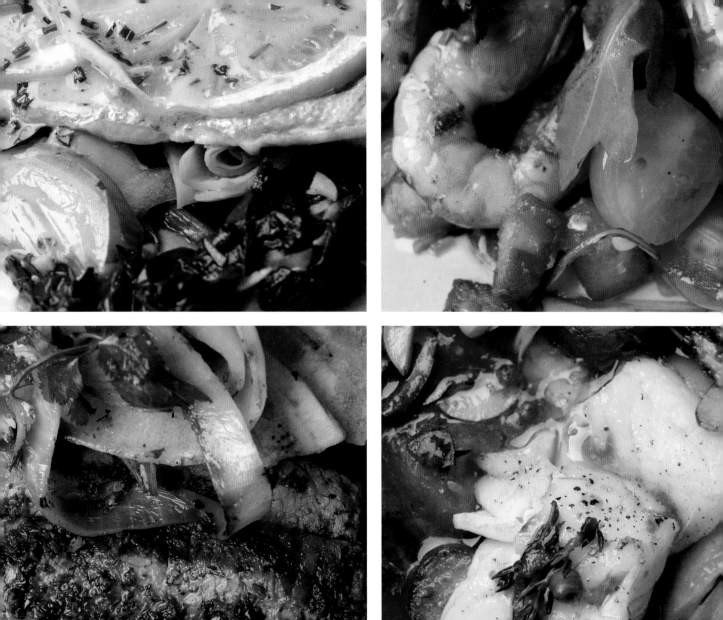
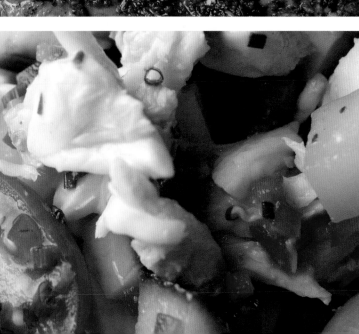
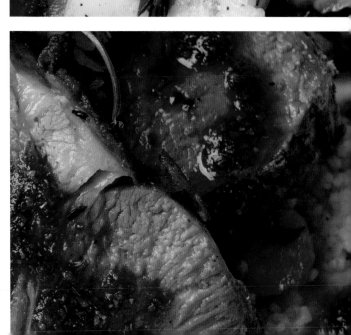

Dinner The Menu

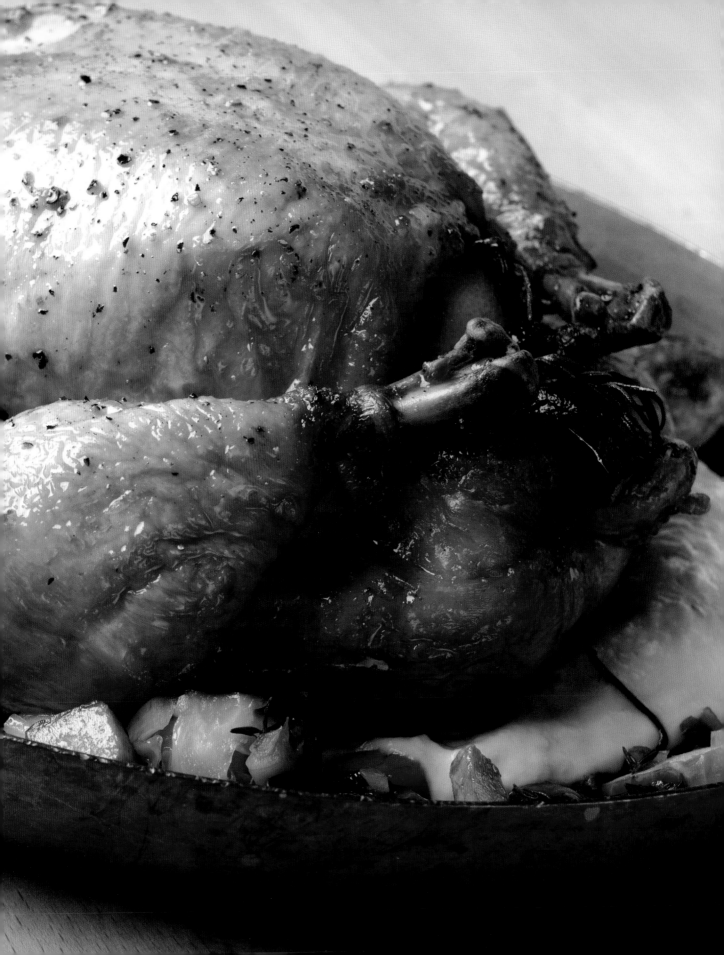

Roast Chicken,
Vegetables & Parsnip Purée
Rediscover the classic chicken dinner—with a 5-star twist.

AS DISCUSSED IN THE NUTRITION CHAPTER, chicken is one of the most important foods to buy organic. If at all possible, try to get to know your farmer and his or her methods. Once you've tasted the alternative to factory-raised meat of any kind, you'll actually become addicted—the difference is just as stark as the methods used to raise the animals.

One big plus of this dish: the parsnips. Parsnips may not have made any trendy superfood list just yet, but it's only a matter of time. In addition to their fiber content (6 grams per cup), they're loaded with potassium, vitamin C, and folate, the last of which can lower your risk for heart disease as well as depression.

What separates this Roast Chicken dinner from a flavor standpoint is the aromatic combination of fresh herbs, garlic, shallots, and vegetables. The kicker is the Parsnip Purée, which surely beats the hell out of any regular gravy you might have otherwise served with the chicken.

The Macros

508
Calories

37g
Protein

15g
Fat

63g
Carbs

Ideal for: Any Day
Makes 6 Servings

+ YOU'LL NEED

For the Roast Chicken:
1 five-pound whole chicken, organic, pasture-raised

1 bunch thyme

1 bunch rosemary

2 lemons, halved

4 cloves garlic

1 tbsp grapeseed oil

Salt and pepper

For the Vegetables:
3 cups brussels sprouts, blanched and halved

1 butternut squash, peeled, diced large

1 shallot, minced

1 tsp garlic, minced

1 tsp fresh thyme, chopped

Juice of 1 lemon

Drizzle of grapeseed oil

1 tbsp honey

1 tsp salt

1 tsp white pepper

For the Sauce:
3 tbsp all-purpose flour

1 cup chicken stock

½ cup demi-glace

For the Parsnip Purée:
8 parsnips, peeled and rough cut

1 qt milk

Salt

White pepper

1 tsp salted butter

+ TO MAKE IT

Roast Chicken:
1 Preheat oven to 350°. Rinse chicken and dry well with paper towels.

2 Stuff cavity of chicken with whole herbs, lemon halves, and garlic cloves. Rub outside of chicken with grapeseed oil and season with salt and pepper.

3 Place chicken on a roasting rack on a sheet pan; this will keep bottom of chicken from burning. Roast for 1¾ hours. Internal temperature should reach 160°.

4 While chicken is roasting, prep vegetables.

Vegetables:
1 Place brussels sprouts, butternut squash, shallot, garlic, chopped thyme, lemon juice, grapeseed oil, honey, salt, and white pepper in a mixing bowl and toss well.

2 Near end of chicken's cooking time, put vegetables on a sheet pan and place in 350° oven for 20–30 minutes, until tender.

Sauce:
When chicken is done, put drippings in a saucepan over medium heat. Add flour, stir well, then add chicken stock and demi-glace. Cook and stir for 3 minutes. Set aside.

Parsnip Purée:
1 Boil parsnips in milk until cooked, 15–20 minutes. Use a colander to strain them, setting milk aside (you may need it for Step 2).

2 Using a food processor or high-performance blender, purée parsnips to a mashed potato-like consistency. Use milk if needed to thin out. Season with salt and white pepper.

To Finish:
Plate with purée first, placing vegetables and chicken on top. Serve sauce on the side.

Roast Trout
with Artichokes &
Charred Lemon
Vinaigrette
A fit fillet.

JUST 3 OUNCES OF TROUT contains 23 grams of protein and only 7 grams of fat. In this recipe, I pair it with Swiss chard, another under-the-radar superfood that's loaded with at least 13 powerful antioxidants. Artichokes, meanwhile, are low-calorie (53 calories per 100 grams) and contain cynarin and sesquiterpene lactones, both of which inhibit the absorption of cholesterol, lowering total cholesterol levels.

As for the taste, I'd be shocked if this didn't become one of your favorite recipes in this book. It's a rare treat when you can pack this many complex, savory flavors into a dish this healthy.

Ideal for: Any Day
Makes 4 Servings

+ YOU'LL NEED

For the Vinaigrette:

3 lemons

1 tbsp white wine vinegar

1 oz honey

1 tbsp extra-virgin olive oil

2 tbsp grapeseed oil

Salt and pepper

½ bunch thyme

For the Trout & Artichokes:

4 trout fillets, 7 oz each

2 tbsp grapeseed oil

12 sliced lemon "wheels"

½ cup red onion, julienned

½ tsp garlic, minced

1 cup artichoke hearts, minced

2 qts Swiss chard, cleaned

1 tsp chives, chopped

1 tsp tarragon, chopped

1 tsp parsley, chopped

Salt and pepper

+ TO MAKE IT

Vinaigrette:

1 Cut lemons in half and grill until nearly blackened on all sides. Place in a covered container and allow to steam for about 5 minutes.

2 Let lemons cool, then juice and zest them.

3 In a blender, add lemon juice, zest, vinegar, and honey. With blender on low, slowly add oils until emulsified. Finish with salt, pepper, and thyme.

Trout & Artichokes:

1 Preheat oven to 350°.

2 Place fish on an oiled sheet pan, skin-side up. Drizzle with a little grapeseed oil and season with salt and pepper. Arrange three thin slices of lemon atop each fillet. Place pan in oven and cook for 8–10 minutes, until done.

3 Heat a large sauté pan over medium-high heat and add 2 tbsp grapeseed oil.

4 Sauté red onions, garlic, and artichokes. Add Swiss chard and deglaze pan with vinaigrette. Once Swiss chard is wilted, remove from heat, season with salt and pepper, and add herbs.

To Finish:

Place Swiss chard and artichokes in the middle of the plate and place trout on top. Spoon extra vinaigrette from pan on top of and around fish.

The Macros

598
Calories

51g
Protein

35g
Fat

20g
Carbs

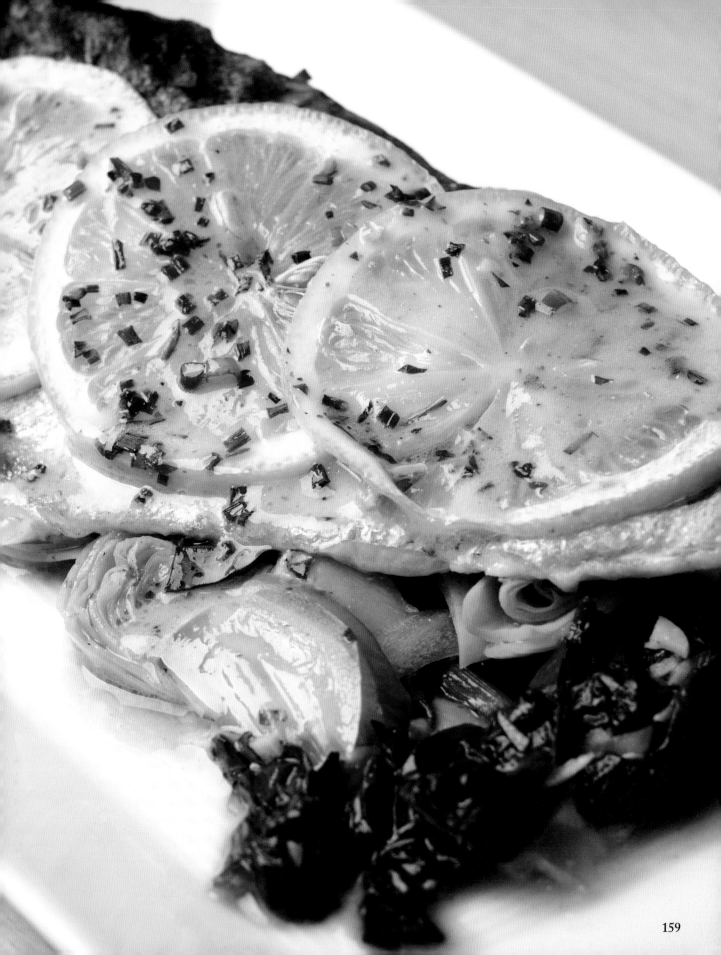

Chilled Crab Salad

A foodie's salad for any night of the week.

LIGHT AND FLAVORFUL, bitter but sweet, with a diverse array of textures, this Chilled Crab Salad is a home run in every sense. To pull it off properly, you need fresh, high-quality ingredients, but assembling the final dish is a cinch.

Crab has an awesome protein-to-fat ratio (about 18:1), which makes it one of my favorite protein sources to cook with. You'll notice the fat content of this recipe is bumped up a little bit, but a lot of that comes from avocado, which has been shown to lower triglyceride and cholesterol levels. Crab is so much more than protein: It's also one of the richest whole-food sources of vitamin B12, which promotes healthy nervous system function and protects you from nerve damage. There's a slight sodium concern with crabmeat—every 3-ounce serving contains more than 900 mg—but since this recipe divides a cup of crabmeat among 4 servings, that shouldn't deter you.

Ideal for: Any Day
Makes 4 Servings

+ YOU'LL NEED

For the Dressing:

¼ **cup** orange juice

2 **tbsp** lemon juice

¼ **cup** champagne vinegar

2 **tsp** Dijon mustard

1 shallot, minced

1 **tsp** honey

Salt

¼ avocado, scooped out

2 **tbsp** grapeseed oil

For the Salad:

½ **cup** grapefruit chunks

½ **cup** green peas

½ **cup** cucumber, minced

1 **tsp** jalapeño, minced

1 mango, diced

1 **tsp** mint, chopped

1 **tsp** chives, chopped

½ **cup** grape tomatoes, halved

¾ avocado, diced

1 bunch watercress tips

1 **cup** jumbo lump crabmeat

+ TO MAKE IT

Dressing:
Purée all dressing ingredients except avocado and oil. Slowly add oil and avocado into blender until smooth. Don't overblend, or dressing will turn dark.

Salad:
Place all salad ingredients except crabmeat in a mixing bowl. Toss well and season with salt and pepper. Gently toss in crabmeat without breaking up lumps. Add dressing and toss until salad is coated.

To Finish:
Divide salad into four martini glasses (for a classy presentation) or four salad bowls.

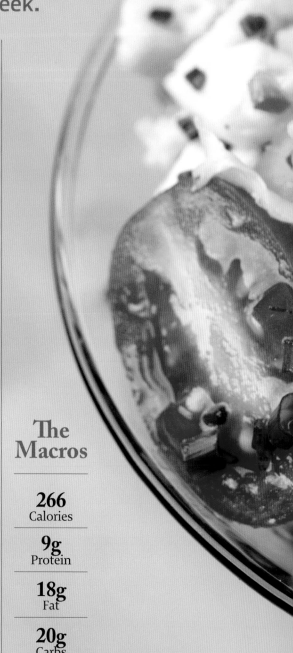

The Macros

266
Calories

9g
Protein

18g
Fat

20g
Carbs

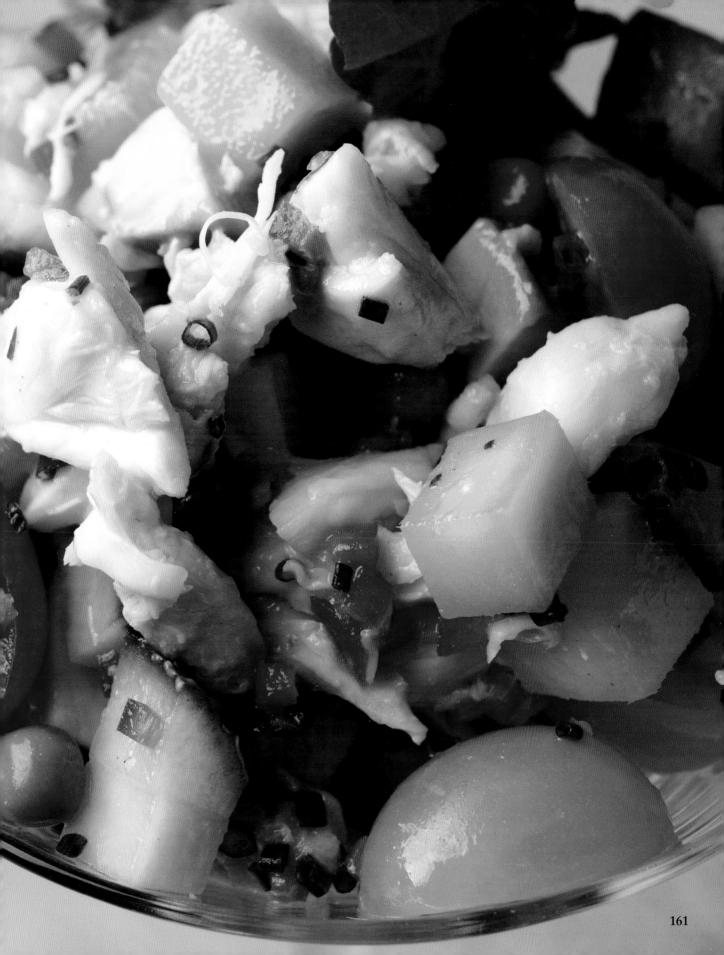

Farro Aubergine

A vegetarian option that doesn't skimp on protein.

LOOK AT ANY BODYBUILDER'S MEAL PLAN, and you're going to notice the same three or four carb sources popping up over and over: rice, sweet potatoes, quinoa, and oatmeal. That's fine in terms of muscle growth, but very limiting for the palate. The list ignores one of the most protein-rich grains on the planet, an ancient grain called farro. Farro is a form of wheat that has a rich, nutty taste and packs 8 grams of protein per cup, as well as 8 grams of fiber.

In this dish, I pair farro with roasted eggplant (aubergine) for a meal that can stand on its own as a vegetarian option, or be paired with a lean meat of your choice for an extra shot of protein.

Ideal for: Any Day
Makes 6 Servings

+ YOU'LL NEED

3 eggplant

3 tbsp extra-virgin olive oil

Salt and pepper

2 cups farro

2 cloves garlic

1 bay leaf

5 cups low-sodium vegetable stock

1 cup balsamic vinegar

1 tsp honey

1 cup red onions, diced small

1 cup red peppers, diced small

1 cup yellow peppers, diced small

1 cup asparagus, blanched

4 oz low-sodium vegetable broth

1 bunch parsley, chopped

6 oz goat cheese, crumbled

+ TO MAKE IT

Eggplant:

1 Preheat oven to 350°.

2 Cut eggplant in half lengthwise and trim off enough of the rounded sides to allow sliced eggplant to sit firmly, faceup, on a plate. Drizzle with olive oil and season with salt and pepper.

3 On a grill or in a broiler, grill eggplant on both sides and place on a sheet pan. Finish in oven for 15–20 minutes, until tender; remove and let cool.

Farro:

1 In a heated saucepan, add 2 tbsp olive oil and farro. Toast for 1 minute.

2 Add garlic, bay leaf, and vegetable stock and bring to a simmer. Turn heat down low and allow farro to cook for 25–30 minutes, until slightly tender.

3 Strain excess liquid from cooked farro and spread farro out on a sheet pan to cool.

Balsamic Reduction:

1 In a small pot over medium heat, slowly reduce balsamic vinegar by two-thirds.

2 Remove reduction from heat and stir in honey. Allow to cool to room temperature before using.

To Finish:

1 Heat a large sauté pan over medium-high heat and add 1 tbsp olive oil. Add diced red onion and red and yellow peppers.

2 Lightly season with salt and pepper and continue to sauté until red onions are translucent.

3 Add asparagus and farro. Deglaze with vegetable stock and continue to cook for 2 minutes to allow farro to absorb stock. Finish with chopped parsley and set aside.

4 Place ½ eggplant in the center of the plate. (You can warm eggplant up quickly in the oven beforehand.) Mount warm farro salad on top of each eggplant. Garnish by lightly drizzling balsamic reduction on top and around eggplant. Finish by topping with crumbled goat cheese.

The Macros

374 Calories

16g Protein

18g Fat

44g Carbs

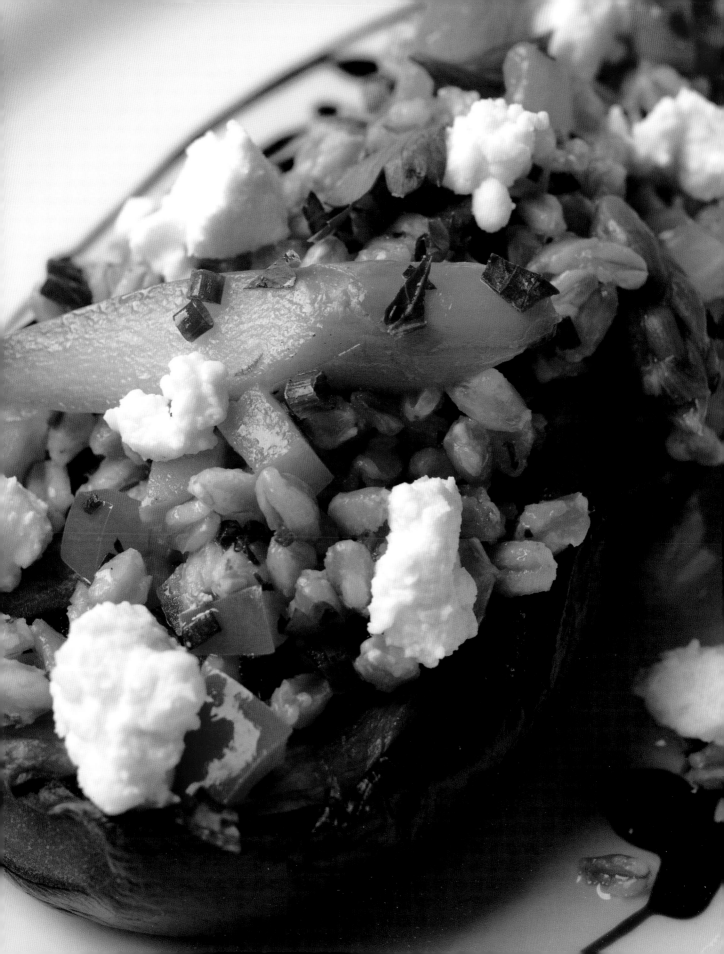

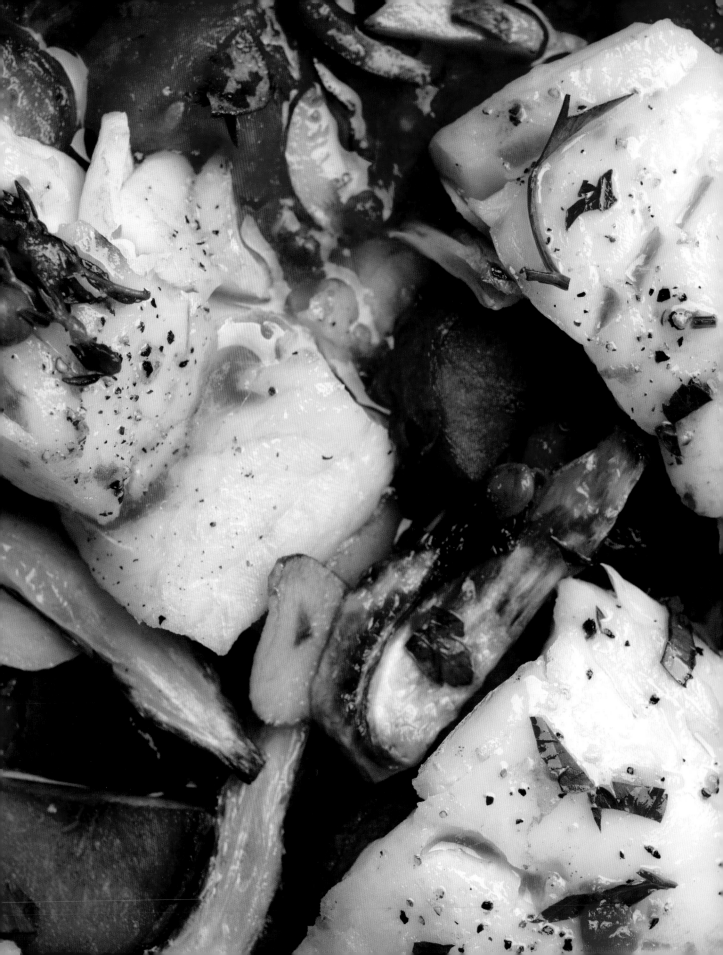

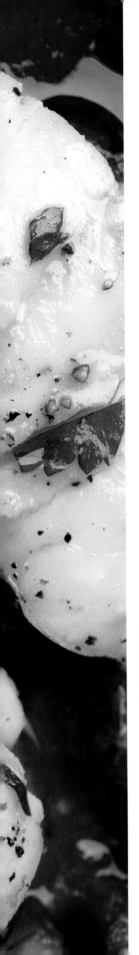

Provençal Roasted Halibut

A smart dieter's secret weapon.

FOR ANYONE TRYING TO LOSE WEIGHT or stay lean, fish is always a good option. If you count yourself in that category and also find cravings so hard to fight that you typically call a meal "done" when your stomach is fit to burst, I'd recommend you put halibut at the top of your list. A meaty white fish, halibut is simultaneously dense, or "heavy," yet low in calories and high in protein.

The French Provençal accompaniment of Niçoise olives, garlic, and San Marzano tomatoes (the best plum tomatoes around; use regular plum tomatoes if you can't find them) builds a rich flavor that adds to the satisfying nature of the halibut.

Even if you're trying to cut weight, you can go back for seconds without derailing your entire diet.

The Macros

599
Calories

57g
Protein

14g
Fat

72g
Carbs

Ideal for: Any Day
Makes 4 Servings

+ YOU'LL NEED

1 tbsp grapeseed oil

4 halibut fillets, 7 oz each

Salt and pepper

16 San Marzano plum tomatoes, whole, peeled

1 large bulb fennel, thinly julienned

4 cloves garlic, thinly sliced

16 sprigs thyme

12 sprigs oregano, roughly chopped

4 tsp capers

12 baby Yukon Gold potatoes, cooked and sliced

32 Niçoise olives, pitted

½ bunch parsley, finely chopped

+ TO MAKE IT

1 Preheat oven to 375°.

2 Add grapeseed oil to a sauté pan over medium-high heat. Season fish with salt and pepper and sear on both sides, until golden brown.

3 Across bottom of a casserole dish, arrange tomatoes, fennel, garlic, thyme, oregano, capers, potatoes, and olives. Place fish on top.

4 Slightly cover fish with vegetables. Ladle olives over fish and place in oven. Allow to cook for 15–20 minutes, until fish is done and vegetables have slightly caramelized.

5 Take dish out of oven and drain off most of the oil. Garnish with chopped parsley and serve family-style.

Seared Wild Salmon
with Green Curry The flavor is untamed.

THERE ARE are several notable health benefits to using wild versus farmed salmon: Wild salmon contains more iron, potassium, and zinc—yet just about *half* the fat of farm-raised salmon. To find wild salmon, you'll need to call ahead to fish markets in your area to be certain they're carrying it, but it's worth the trouble.

The black rice, sometimes called forbidden rice, adds carbs that hit the spot with even more iron, vitamin E, and a payload of antioxidants that would rival any other so-called superfood. The Green Curry Sauce, made with coconut milk, mirin wine (a rice wine similar to sake), cilantro, and garlic adds an elegant layer of savory spices that create a memorable meal you'll come back to time and again.

Ideal for: A Hard Training Day
Makes 4 Servings

+ YOU'LL NEED

For the Rice:

1 cup black rice

1 tsp grapeseed oil

1 tsp fresh thyme, chopped

Salt

1 bay leaf

3¼ cups chicken stock

For the Green Curry Sauce:

¼ cup onion, diced small

1 clove garlic, minced

1 tbsp grapeseed oil

Salt and pepper

½ cup mirin wine

6 oz coconut milk

3 tbsp rice wine vinegar

3 tbsp green curry paste

¼ bunch cilantro sprigs

For the Salmon &
Clams or Cockles:

2 tbsp grapeseed oil

4 wild salmon fillets, 7 oz each

20 petite clams or cockles

2 tbsp mirin wine

1 tsp garlic, minced

1 tsp ginger, minced

1 tsp scallion, minced

1 lime, halved

1 tbsp salted butter

20 sprigs cilantro

Salt and pepper

+ TO MAKE IT

Rice:

1 In a rondo (a wide, shallow pot) over high heat, toast rice with oil, thyme, salt, and bay leaves for 3 minutes. Add 3 cups of the chicken stock and cook on medium-low heat for 20–30 minutes, until done.

2 Turn off heat and let rice rest for 10 minutes before removing from pot.

Green Curry Sauce:

1 In a medium saucepan over high heat, sauté onions and garlic with grapeseed oil, salt, and pepper. Once onions are translucent, add mirin wine to deglaze, then add coconut milk, rice wine vinegar, and curry paste.

2 Whisk ingredients together and simmer for 2–3 minutes. Remove from heat and add cilantro sprigs. Blend until a sauce forms.

3 Season with salt and pepper. Don't keep too hot; this will cause it to discolor.

Salmon & Clams or Cockles:

1 Add 1 tbsp grapeseed oil to a hot sauté pan. Once hot, add salmon and sear for 2–3 minutes. Turn salmon over (when it's ready to be turned, it won't stick to the pan) and continue to cook for 3–4 minutes, until done.

2 For clams or cockles: Add 1 tbsp grapeseed oil to a hot sauté pan. Add clams or cockles, garlic, ginger, and scallions. Deglaze pan with mirin wine.

3 Add Curry Sauce and cover pan to allow clams to steam open.

4 Once clams have opened (discard any that don't open) add lime juice and butter. Continue to reduce clams in sauce until butter has melted.

To Finish:

1 Reheat rice with a small amount of chicken stock to make it hot and moist.

2 Add a mound of rice in the center of a large plate or shallow entrée bowl. Ladle some curry sauce around rice. Arrange clams or cockles around rice and place fish on top. Garnish with cilantro.

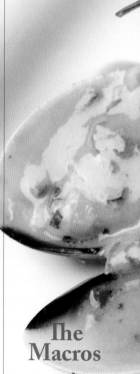

The Macros

752
Calories

48g
Protein

40g
Fat

54g
Carbs

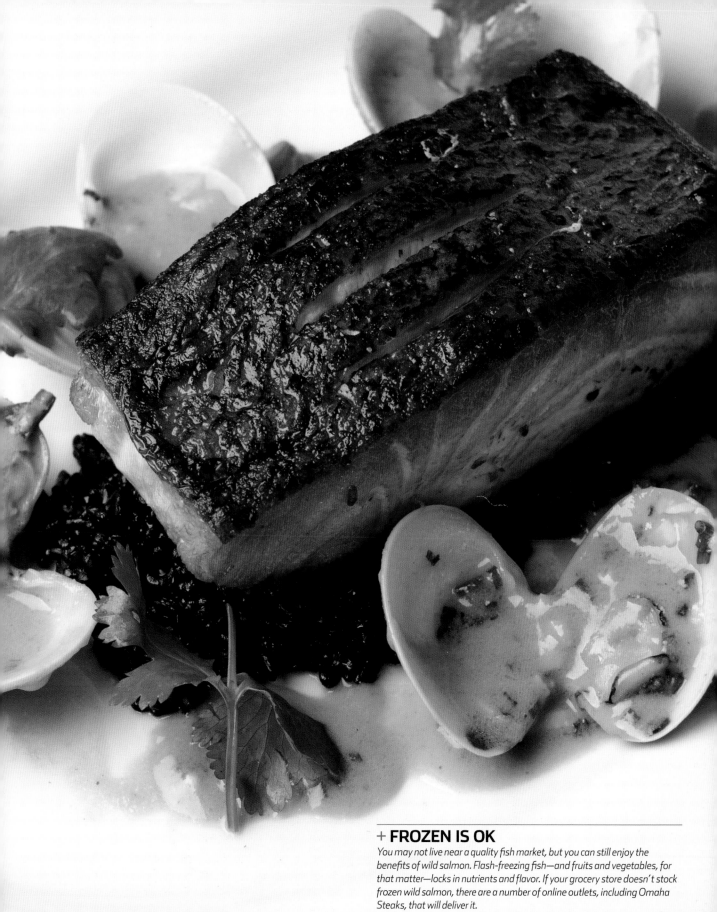

+ FROZEN IS OK

You may not live near a quality fish market, but you can still enjoy the benefits of wild salmon. Flash-freezing fish—and fruits and vegetables, for that matter—locks in nutrients and flavor. If your grocery store doesn't stock frozen wild salmon, there are a number of online outlets, including Omaha Steaks, that will deliver it.

Grilled Cuban Steak
with Cilantro Chimichurri
& Crispy Plantain Chips

Everything has its place—even juicy red meat with fried plantains.

CUBAN CUISINE IS A UNIQUE, SPICY COLLISION of Latin and African influences. While immensely enjoyable, too many Cuban dishes are needlessly heavy plates of arroz con pollo (chicken and rice), fatty steak, and fried plantains.

But there's a way you can enjoy these eclectic Cuban flavors—preferably on a cheat day—without the meal becoming a massive belly bomb. In this Grilled Cuban Steak recipe, we'll use flank steak, a lean cut of beef that will stay tender if you keep it on the medium-rare side, and Cilantro Chimichurri, which will help keep it moist.

You can also enjoy those infamous plantain chips. Though similar to bananas, plantains actually contain more potassium and vitamins A and C than bananas. When lightly fried in grapeseed oil then drained of the excess, plantains make a delectable side dish— they're sweet but not overly so, and add a satisfying crunch.

Ideal for: A Cheat Day
Makes 6 Servings

+ YOU'LL NEED

For the Chimichurri:
1 bunch cilantro
1 bunch parsley
1 dash crushed red pepper
¼ **cup** grapeseed oil
Juice of **3** lemons
Zest of **1** lemon
2 tbsp red wine vinegar
¼ **cup** water

For the Plantain Chips:
3 green plantains, peeled and thinly sliced
2 tbsp grapeseed oil
Salt and pepper

For the Dry Rub:
2 tsp cumin powder
2 tsp paprika
½ **tsp** garlic powder
1 tsp crushed red pepper
1 tsp Cajun seasoning
1 tsp salt

For the Steak:
3 lbs grass-fed Angus flank steak
1 large Vidalia onion, sliced into ½-inch-thick rings
Salt and pepper
2 tbsp grapeseed oil
12 lime wedges
½ bunch cilantro sprigs

+ TO MAKE IT

Chimichurri:
Place all chimichurri ingredients into a blender and purée until almost smooth.

Plantain Chips:
1 Preheat oven to 350°.

2 Toss plantain slices with oil and arrange in a single layer on a sheet pan. Season with salt and pepper.

3 Bake for 20–25 minutes, until light golden brown.

4 When plantains come out of oven, place them on paper towels to drain.

Steak:
1 Preheat grill to medium-high heat. Combine all Dry Rub ingredients in a bowl, then rub mixture on both sides of steak.

2 Brush sliced onions with grapeseed oil and season with salt and pepper.

3 Place steak on grill and cook each side for 4–6 minutes, to desired doneness.

4 Add onions to grill when meat is almost done. Grill onions on both sides; handle gingerly to avoid breaking them.

5 Once steak and onions are done, let steak rest. Put onions in a mixing bowl. Squeeze 6 lime wedges on top of onions. Add half of the cilantro sprigs and season with salt and pepper. Set aside.

To Finish:
1 Slice steak on a bias and arrange on a large platter.

2 Scatter warm grilled onions on top of steak. Drizzle with chimichurri and garnish with plantain chips and remaining cilantro sprigs and lime wedges.

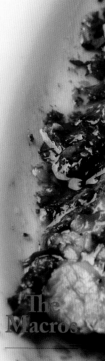

The Macros

781
Calories

65g
Protein

50g
Fat

14g
Carbs

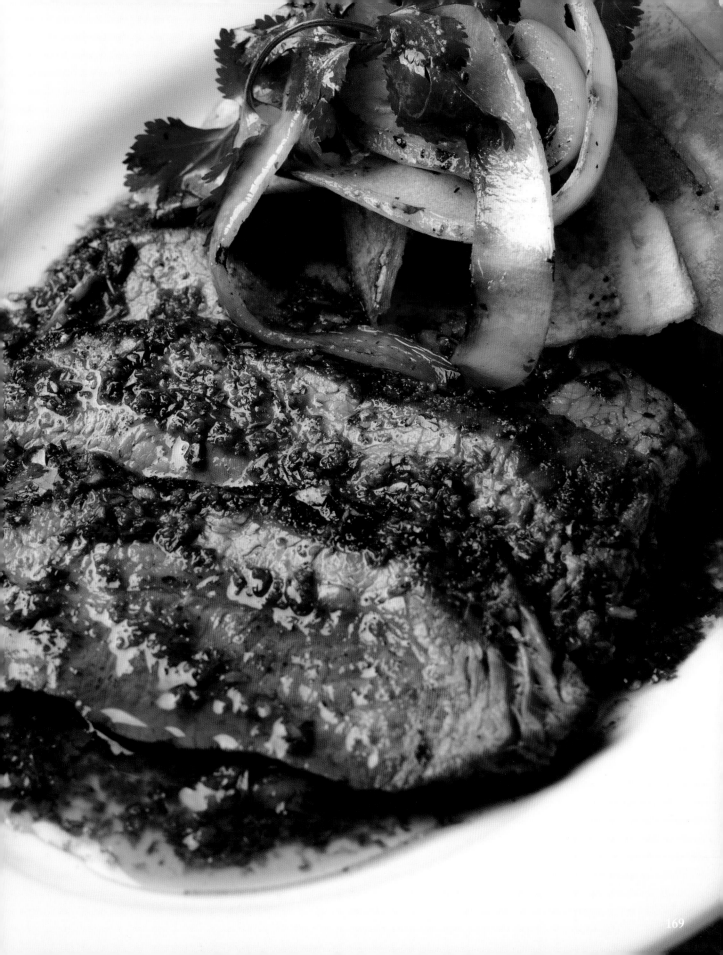

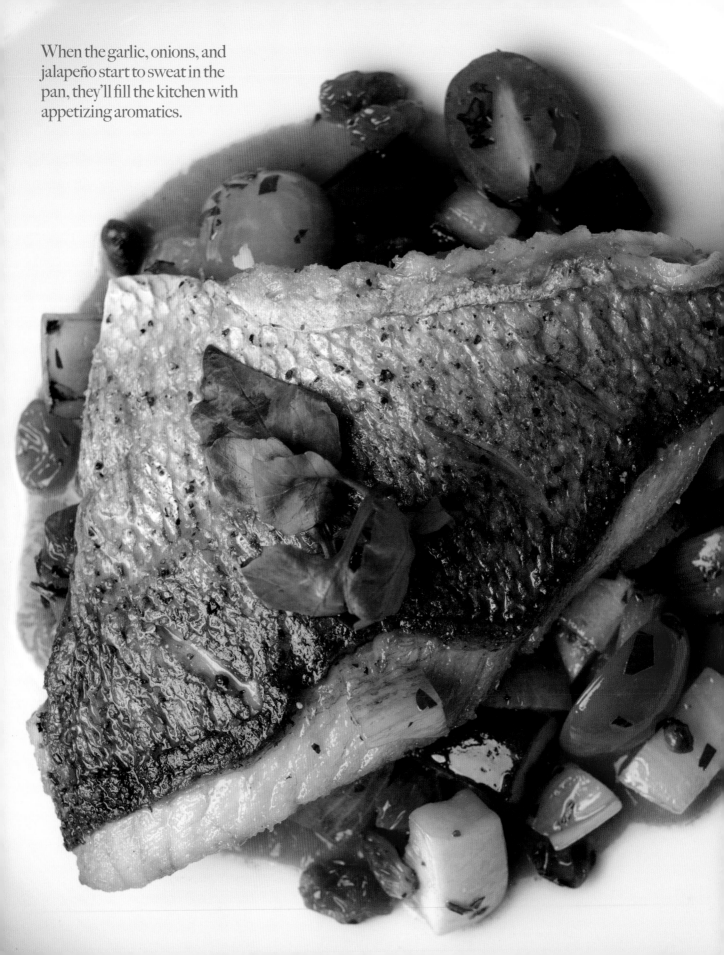

When the garlic, onions, and jalapeño start to sweat in the pan, they'll fill the kitchen with appetizing aromatics.

Mediterranean Sea Bass
with Catalán Sauce
So good for you, second helpings are encouraged.

THERE'S ONE GOLDEN RULE when it comes to vegetables: The more you eat, the better. We could debate the benefits of organic and non-GMO all day, but the most essential fact you need to retain is that no matter how many vegetables you think you're eating, you're probably not eating enough.

I've paired this Mediterranean sea bass (aka branzino) with a simple ratatouille (another name for stewed vegetables), which makes it easy to fill up on the amount and variety of veggies you need. Comprised of zucchini, yellow squash, eggplant, and grape tomatoes—with an aromatic base of garlic, fennel, and red onion—this healthy combo is anything but boring.

The branzino itself is loaded with protein, with 22 grams per 4 ounces, and a meager 3 grams of fat. (Naturally, the final macros vary due to the inclusion of other ingredients in the recipe.) It's light in flavor, which makes it easy to put away more than one serving. Lucky for you, that's not a bad thing.

The Macros

315
Calories

24g
Protein

18g
Fat

13g
Carbs

Ideal for: Any Day
Makes 6 Servings

+ YOU'LL NEED

For the Catalán Sauce:

1 clove garlic

¼ cup onion, diced

¼ jalapeño pepper

1 tsp extra-virgin olive oil

1 red pepper, cleaned of seeds and sliced large

1 tbsp tomato paste

¼ cup white wine

1 cup 1% milk

Juice of ¼ lemon

Salt

For the Sea Bass & Ratatouille:

2 tbsp grapeseed oil

½ cup red onion, diced large

½ cup fennel, diced large

1 cup zucchini, diced large

1 cup yellow squash, diced large

1 cup eggplant, peeled and diced large

½ cup grape tomatoes

2 cloves garlic, slivered

¼ cup white wine

1 tbsp capers

2 tbsp golden raisins

½ cup tomato sauce

4 branzino fillets, 6 oz. each, skin on

+ TO MAKE IT

Catalán Sauce:

1 In a sauté pan over medium heat, sweat the garlic, onions, and jalapeño in oil. Add red pepper and cook briefly. Add tomato paste, deglaze with white wine, and reduce for 3 minutes.

2 Add milk and reduce sauce by one-third. Purée in a high-performance blender until very smooth, and season with lemon juice and salt.

Sea Bass & Ratatouille:

1 Heat a large sauté pan and add 3 tbsp grapeseed oil. Add red onion and fennel and sauté for 2–3 minutes. Add zucchini, yellow squash, eggplant, tomatoes, and garlic. Continue to sauté veggies until tender. Deglaze pan with white wine, and add capers, raisins, and tomato sauce. Season with salt and pepper.

2 Heat a large sauté pan and add 3 tbsp grapeseed oil. Once hot, add fish and sear skin-side down. When all skin is golden brown and crispy, turn fish over using a fish spatula. Continue to cook for 2 more minutes.

To Finish:

Ladle 3 tbsp sauce into the center of the plate and swirl around to create a circle of sauce. Place a tight portion of ratatouille in the center of the sauce. Arrange fish on top of veggies and serve.

Seared Sea Scallops
with White Bean Sofrito

Lean protein, high fiber, and enough complexity to satisfy any palate.

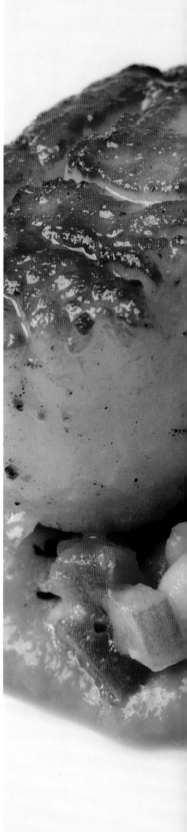

SCALLOPS OFFER THE SAME BENEFITS as other seafood—high protein, omega-3 fats, magnesium, potassium. They also offer plenty that's unique: Their mild, sweet flavor and soft fleshy texture typically win over people who don't like other forms of shellfish. This is especially important if you have a fussy eater in the family.

The White Bean Sofrito (a base sauce used in many Latin dishes) boosts the protein and fiber content, and the English Sweet Pea Purée adds a creamy sweetness that perfectly balances the dish.

Ideal for: Any Day
Makes 4 Servings

+ YOU'LL NEED

For the English Sweet Pea Purée:

1½ cups English sweet peas, blanched

1 cup chicken stock, cold

1 oz honey

1 tsp salt

1 dash white pepper

For the White Bean Sofrito:

6 shallots, minced

2 oz extra-virgin olive oil

2 red peppers, brunoised (julienned, then cross-cut)

1 cup white wine

2 cups white beans, cooked

2 oz lemon juice

Chicken stock, as needed

1 pat salted butter

Salt and pepper

For the Sea Scallops:

2 tbsp grapeseed oil

16 U-10* dry sea scallops

Salt and pepper

+ TO MAKE IT

English Sweet Pea Purée:
Place sweet peas in a high-performance blender. Blend slowly and add chicken stock and honey. Blend faster and add salt and white pepper. Continue until very smooth.

White Bean Sofrito:
In a sauté pan over medium heat, sweat the shallots in olive oil, then add peppers. Cook for 1 minute, then deglaze with white wine. Add beans, lemon juice, a small splash of chicken stock, and butter.

Sea Scallops:
In a large sauté pan over medium-high heat, add 3 tbsp grapeseed oil. Once hot, add scallops and cook for 2–3 minutes on each side, until golden brown.

To Finish:
Place a spoonful of purée on the plate and pull a tablespoon across it from left to right. Add sofrito in center of purée and place 4 scallops on top of beans.

The Macros

568
Calories

38g
Protein

24g
Fat

43g
Carbs

*Large scallops. It would take fewer than 10 of this size to add up to a pound.

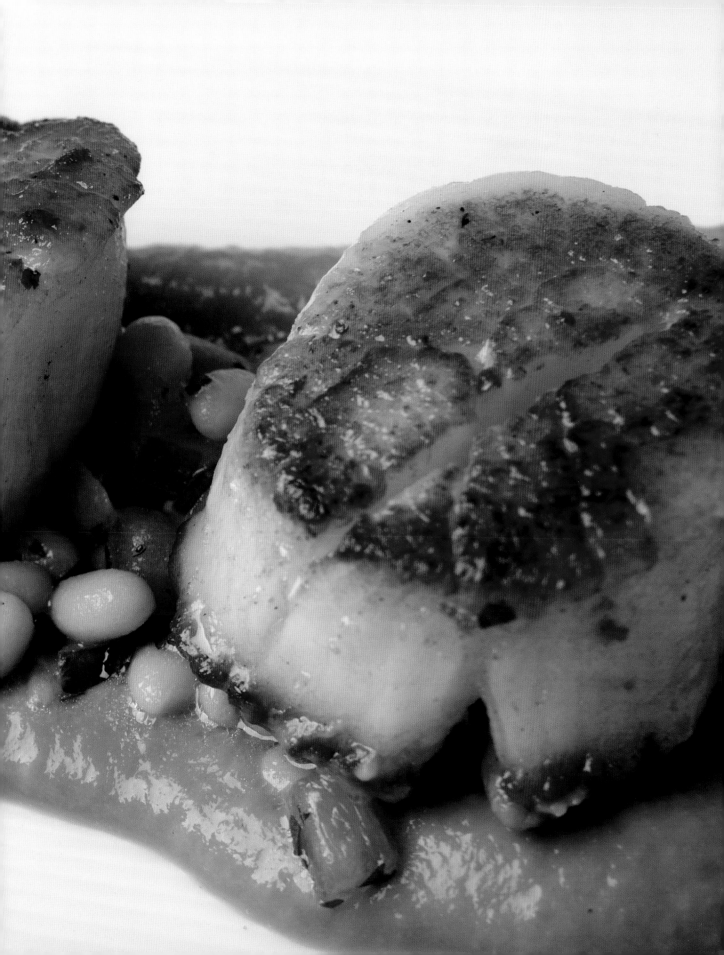

Tuna au Poivre

Spicy and mouthwatering: Heart-friendly food never tasted so good.

A GENEROUS HELPING OF SPICE makes any food more satisfying. Here, that spice comes in the form of the green peppercorns in the Au Poivre Sauce and the crushed black pepper, mustard, and fennel seeds used to form a crust on the tuna. Be sure not to overcook the tuna; since we're using ahi tuna, it's best eaten rare to medium-rare or you risk losing the melt-in-your-mouth texture and flavor. Don't cook it more than 3–4 minutes per side over medium-high heat. Overcooked tuna will be dry and relatively flavorless.

On top of the heart-health benefits offered by the omega-3s in tuna, one recent study found that people who eat fish at least five times a week can lower their risk of stroke by up to 52%.

Ideal for: A Hard Training Day
Makes 6 Servings

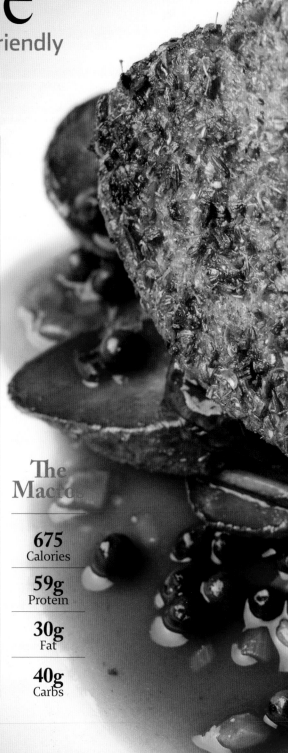

+ YOU'LL NEED

For the Au Poivre Sauce:

1 shallot, minced

1 tbsp green peppercorns in brine

1 bay leaf

1 tsp salted butter

3 tbsp brandy

1 cup demi-glace

¼ cup heavy cream

1 tsp lemon juice

Salt

For the Tuna:

5 tbsp grapeseed oil

2 cups baby Yukon Gold potatoes, blanched and cut in half

1 lb fresh spinach

6 tbsp black peppercorns, crushed

3 tbsp mustard seed, crushed

3 tbsp fennel seed, crushed

6 ahi tuna steaks, 6 oz each

Salt

+ TO MAKE IT

Au Poivre Sauce:
In a sauté pan over medium heat, sauté shallots, green peppercorns, and bay leaf in butter for 1 minute. Deglaze pan with brandy, then add demi-glace and heavy cream. Reduce by three-quarters, add lemon juice, and season with salt.

Tuna:
1 Heat a large sauté pan over medium heat and add 2 tbsp of the grapeseed oil. Add potatoes and allow to brown slightly. Then add spinach and continue to sauté until it's wilted.

2 Heat a large, nonstick sauté pan to high heat and add 3 tbsp grapeseed oil. Combine crushed pepper, mustard, and fennel seeds on a plate and crust all sides of tuna with spices. Season with salt, then sear tuna evenly on each side for about 3 minutes, cooking to medium-rare.

To Finish:
Place a bed of spinach and potatoes in the center of the plate, then spoon sauce around it. Slice one tuna steak in half, and arrange halves on top of spinach and potatoes.

The Macros

675
Calories

59g
Protein

30g
Fat

40g
Carbs

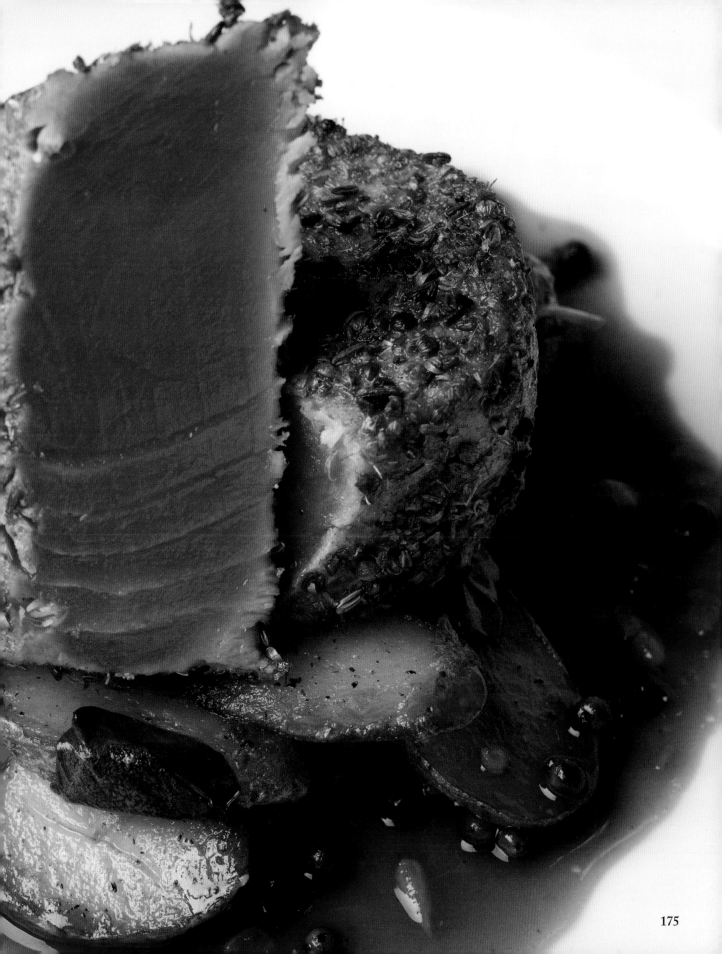

Moroccan Lamb
with Saffron Couscous & Honey-Roasted Carrots

Even a cheat meal needs protein and healthy fats. This is a rich reward that makes sense.

LAMB HAS THE REPUTATION OF BEING A FATTY MEAT—a reputation that's well-deserved in this era of lot-feeding and all-corn diets. But 100% grass-fed (or grass-finished) lamb retains the rich flavor you'd expect, with more of its fat coming from omega-3s as well as conjugated linoleic acid (CLA), which research shows can target belly fat and help burn it faster. It's obvious, then, that you need to go for grass-fed when making this recipe. Have your butcher french the rack of lamb—clean the ends of the bones, so they're exposed—to get a time-consuming step out of the way.

Ideal for: A Cheat Day
Makes 4 Servings

+ YOU'LL NEED

For the Marinade:

1 tbsp thyme, chopped

1 tbsp garlic, minced

1 tbsp ginger, minced

1 tbsp grapeseed oil

1 tsp coriander powder

½ tsp cumin powder

½ tsp fennel seeds

½ tsp paprika powder

Salt and pepper

For the Saffron Couscous:

2 cups chicken broth

1 tsp saffron

3 oz salted butter

¼ tsp salt

1 cup couscous, uncooked

½ cup golden raisins

For the Honey-Roasted Carrots:

2 cups carrots, peeled and diced medium

2 tbsp grapeseed oil

1 dash cumin powder

2 tbsp honey

Salt

For the Harissa
(Hot Chili Pepper Paste):

1 garlic clove

1½ tsp coriander powder

½ cup grapeseed oil

1½ tsp cumin powder

½ tsp fennel seeds

½ tsp caraway seeds, toasted and ground

1½ tsp paprika powder

½ tsp cayenne pepper

½ tsp salt

½ tsp red wine vinegar

For the Lamb:

1 four-bone rack of grass-fed lamb, frenched and trimmed of fat

For the Vegetables:

1 tbsp salted butter

½ cup chicken stock

1 cup green peas

1 cup chickpeas

Salt and pepper

1 tbsp parsley, chopped

+ TO MAKE IT

Marinade:

1 In a mixing bowl, combine all marinade ingredients.

2 At least 30 minutes prior to roasting, place lamb in a roasting pan and pour marinade in, covering lamb as much as possible.

Saffron Couscous:

1 In a saucepan, bring chicken broth to a boil, then add saffron, butter, and salt.

2 Stir in couscous and raisins.

3 Remove saucepan from heat and cover with foil or plastic wrap. Let sit for 5–7 minutes. Couscous should be light and puffy.

Honey-Roasted Carrots:

1 Preheat oven to 350°.

2 Toss all carrot ingredients together in a mixing bowl, then spread carrots over a sheet pan.

3 Roast for 20 minutes, or until tender and lightly caramelized.

Harissa:

1 Purée garlic and oil in a blender.

2 Pour purée into a mixing bowl; add remainder of harissa ingredients and whisk together.

Lamb:

1 Preheat oven to 350°.

2 In a hot sauté pan, sear marinated rack of lamb on all sides and place on a sheet pan with a roasting rack. Roast in oven for 12–15 minutes, until medium-rare. Let lamb rest for 5 minutes before carving.

Vegetables:

In another warm sauté pan, add butter and chicken stock. Once butter is melted into stock, add honey-roasted carrots, green peas, and chickpeas. When veggies are warm, season with salt and pepper, and add parsley.

To Finish:

Arrange couscous, vegetables, and sliced lamb on the plate. Drizzle harissa around plate.

+ HOT ZONE

The harissa—or hot chili pepper paste—in this couscous adds a decisive kick that serves as a nice balance to the richness of the lamb.

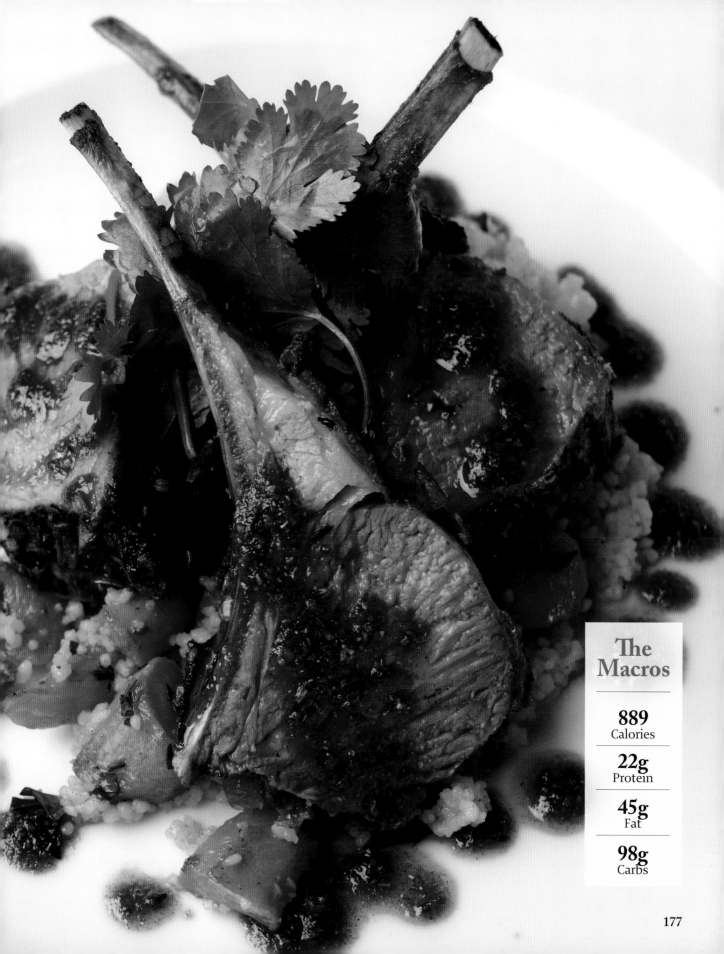

The
Macros

889
Calories

22g
Protein

45g
Fat

98g
Carbs

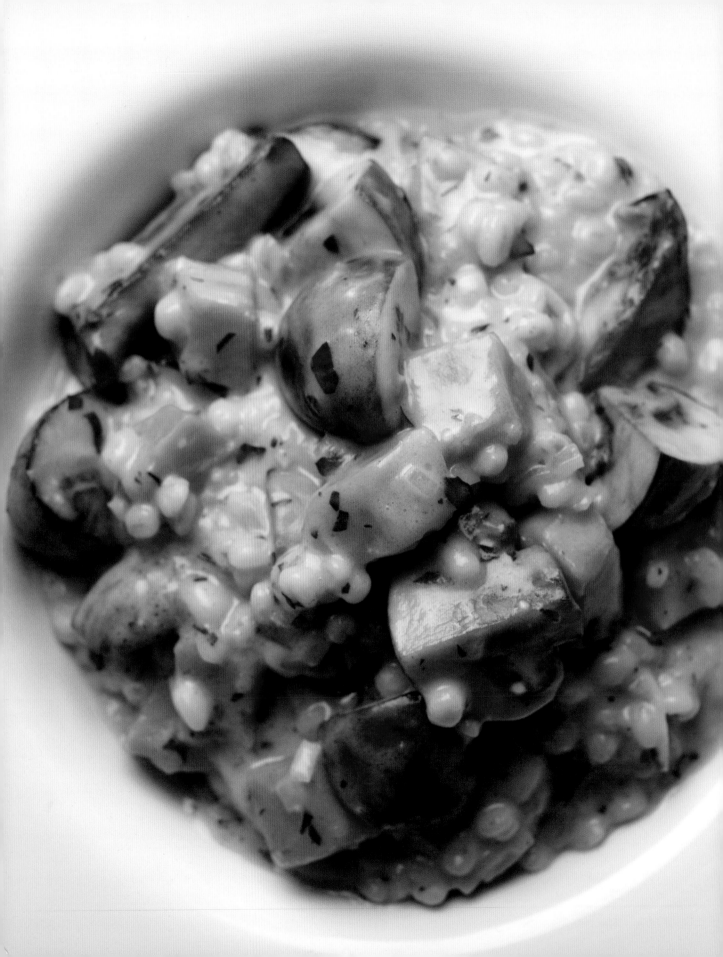

Wild Mushroom & Butternut Barlotto

An essential dish for any mushroom lover.

ONE OF THE GREAT SECRETS ABOUT MUSHROOMS: They're rich in nutrients that have a direct effect on athletic performance. These include selenium, a testosterone booster, and niacin, which increases blood flow to working muscles. Mushrooms are also one of the few non-fortified foods loaded with vitamin D, which is crucial for maintaining muscle efficiency and function.

While the importance of whole grains is well-known, barley—outside of its use in beer—is less recognized as a healthy grain. That's a shame, because it has a robust flavor profile most people would enjoy, and provides healthy complex carbs that can fuel long sessions in the gym. Barley takes center stage in this recipe for barlotto—a risotto-style dish in which the short-grain rice is replaced by pearl barley.

If you need to up the protein content of this meal, feel free to pair it with grilled chicken or serve it as a side dish with another lean meal. Nevertheless, I'm confident you'll see this recipe has the strength to stand on its own.

The Macros

531
Calories

20g
Protein

14g
Fat

78g
Carbs

Ideal for: A Hard Training Day
Makes 6 Servings

+ YOU'LL NEED

For the Barley:

5 cups low-sodium chicken broth

2 cups pearl barley, rinsed

1 bay leaf

For the Squash:

1 medium butternut squash, cleaned

2 tbsp extra-virgin olive oil

Salt and pepper

For the Mushrooms:

3 tbsp extra-virgin olive oil

2 shallots, minced

8 thin slices garlic clove

2 cups maitake mushrooms, sliced

2 cups oyster mushrooms, sliced

2 cups crimini mushrooms, quartered

Salt and pepper

To Finish:

½ cup white wine

2 cups low-sodium chicken broth

½ cup Parmesan cheese, grated

1 tbsp fresh chives, chopped

1 tbsp fresh parsley, chopped

1 tbsp fresh tarragon, chopped

+ TO MAKE IT

Barley:

1 Bring chicken broth to a boil and add rinsed barley and bay leaf.

2 Cook for 30–35 minutes, until slightly al dente.

3 Spread cooked barley on a sheet pan to cool.

Squash:

1 Preheat oven to 350°.

2 Carefully peel squash and cut bottom (round part) off. Cut squash in half and remove seeds, then dice into large pieces.

3 In a large mixing bowl, toss diced squash with oil and salt and pepper. Place on a sheet pan and roast in oven for 15–20 minutes, until tender and slightly caramelized.

Mushrooms:

1 In a large sauté pan over medium-high heat, add olive oil, shallots, and garlic. Sweat the shallots and garlic until fragrant, then add mushrooms.

2 Continue to sauté mushrooms until tender. Season lightly with salt and pepper.

To Finish:

1 Deglaze pan with white wine and add chicken broth and cooked barley. Continue to cook on medium heat.

2 Once barley begins to thicken, add Parmesan cheese and finish with chives, parsley, and tarragon.

3 Serve family-style.

Grilled Prawns
with Summer Tomato-Arugula Salad & Sweet Corn Purée
Big flavor, with no guilt in sight.

LIKE MOST OTHER SEAFOOD, prawns pack a good amount of protein and healthy fats into each serving. Their protein-to-fat ratio is a very robust 15:1, and they have moderate amounts of calcium (for healthy bones) and vitamin E (for healthy skin).

Since there isn't a huge flavor or nutritional difference between prawns and shrimp, you can use them interchangeably in this recipe. The main differences between prawns and shrimp are their size, shape, and texture—elements that all contribute to the overall enjoyment of any meal—so I encourage you to try both and see which you like best. Now the fun part: This dish is a complete knockout—the flavors absolutely kill, and the Sweet Corn Purée makes it as satisfying as any comfort food you can think of.

Ideal for: Any Day
Makes 4 Servings

+ YOU'LL NEED

For the Sweet Corn Purée:

1 oz grapeseed oil

7 ears corn, cooked, kernels cut off

½ Vidalia onion, diced

½ tsp saffron

2 oz vegetable stock

Salt

For the Tomato-Arugula Salad:

½ cup bacon, diced small

1 shallot, minced

1 cup corn, raw, cut from cob

1½ cups red and yellow cherry tomatoes, halved

1 qt baby arugula

Salt and pepper

1 tbsp chives, chopped

Juice of ½ lemon

For the Prawns:

16 prawns, head on; or 16 large shrimp, cleaned

4 tbsp grapeseed oil

Salt and pepper

+ TO MAKE IT

Sweet Corn Purée:

1 Heat 1 oz grapeseed oil in a large sauté pan and add corn and onion. Slowly render (cook through)—do not overcook or caramelize.

2 Add saffron and stir in so color is even.

3 Place mixture in a high-performance blender and purée. Add veggie stock as needed to achieve a thick, smooth purée. Do not overmix or make thin. Season with salt.

Tomato-Arugula Salad:

1 Heat a sauté pan to medium heat and render diced bacon until golden brown. Drain excess fat, then add shallot and corn and continue to cook for 1 minute.

2 Take pan off heat and toss in tomatoes and arugula. Season with salt, pepper, chives, and lemon juice.

Prawns:

1 Preheat grill to medium-high heat.

2 Toss prawns (or shrimp) with 2 tbsp grapeseed oil and salt and pepper.

3 Grill prawns carefully, until golden brown on each side.

To Finish:

Place a spoonful of warm purée in the center of the plate and swirl around to form a circle. Arrange salad in middle of purée, and stack grilled prawns around it.

The Macros

324 Calories

18g Protein

8g Fat

52g Carbs

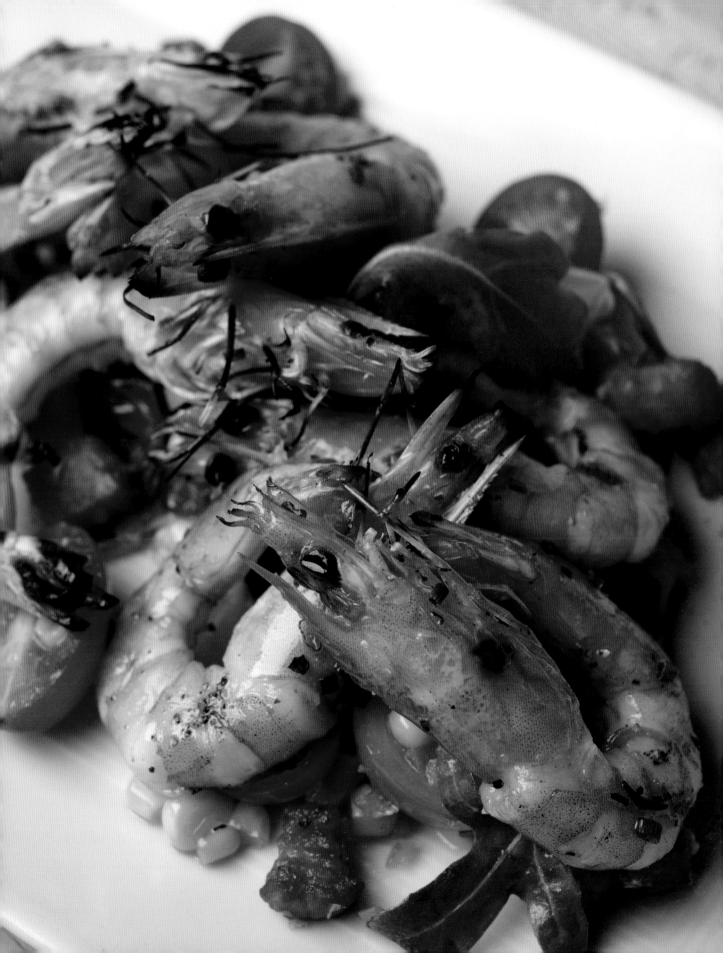

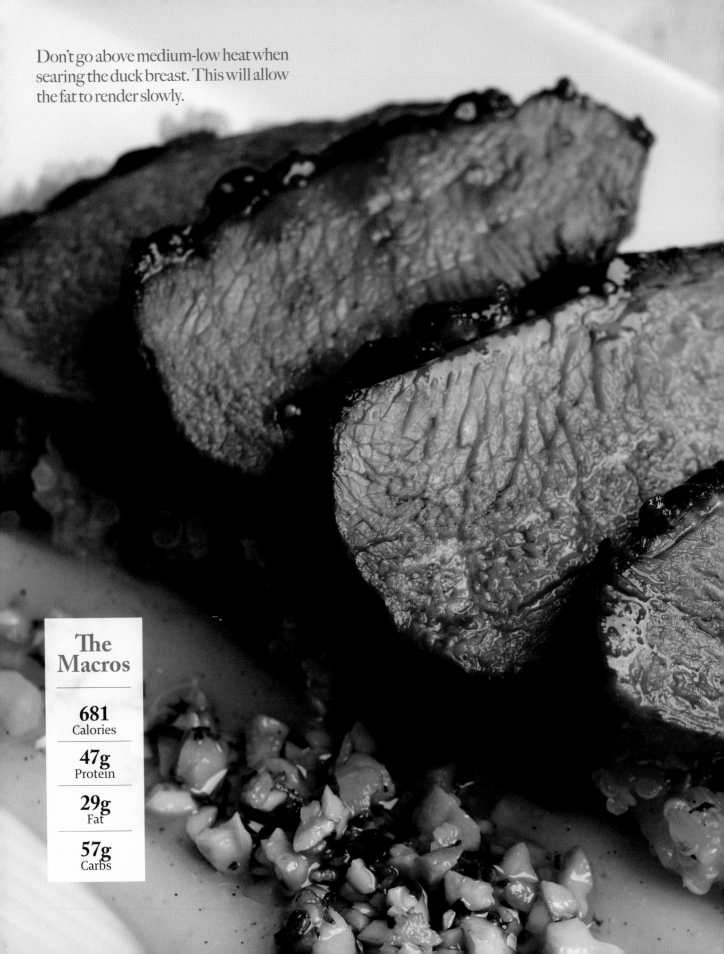

Don't go above medium-low heat when searing the duck breast. This will allow the fat to render slowly.

The Macros

681
Calories

47g
Protein

29g
Fat

57g
Carbs

Fig-Balsamic Glazed Duck Breast

The rich taste of duck, paired with healthy carbs and fats.

ON THE LIST OF LEAN, MUSCLE-BUILDING PROTEINS, duck is near the bottom for most fitness enthusiasts. I understand why: It's fattier than any other poultry, and many recipes call for the skin to be left on while it cooks. It's crispy and delicious, but blows through your daily fat macros in a heartbeat.

But duck's fat content shouldn't outweigh its other benefits. For instance, every 3½-ounce serving packs 18 grams of protein. Duck also contains good amounts of selenium and zinc, two minerals that play a major role in healthy enzyme function and cellular metabolism. It's also rich in vitamin B5, or pantothenic acid, which helps your body make the chemicals needed for nerve signaling.

I also mitigated some of those saturated fat calories by pairing the duck with healthy carbs (from quinoa) and fats (from hazelnuts). A Fig-Balsamic Glaze and Vanilla Pear Purée complete the dish by adding an exciting depth of flavor.

Ideal for: A Hard Training Day
Makes 4 Servings

+ YOU'LL NEED

For the Fig-Balsamic Glaze:
- ½ **cup** dry figs
- 1½ **cups** balsamic vinegar
- 2 **tbsp** honey

For the Pilaf:
- 1 **tbsp** grapeseed oil
- ¼ **cup** celery, minced
- ¼ carrot, minced
- 1 shallot, minced
- 1 **cup** raw quinoa
- 2 **cups** low-sodium chicken broth
- 1 bay leaf

For the Hazelnuts:
- ¼ **cup** hazelnuts, chopped
- 1 sprig rosemary
- 2 **tbsp** grapeseed oil
- 1 clove garlic, minced
- 1 **dash** red pepper flakes
- 1 **tsp** lemon juice

For the Vanilla Pear Purée:
- 4 pears, peeled and cored
- 1 shallot
- 1 vanilla bean
- 1 **tbsp** honey
- 1 **tsp** lemon juice
- 1 **tsp** salted butter

For the Duck:
- 4 duck breasts, 6 oz. each
- Salt and pepper

+ TO MAKE IT

Fig-Balsamic Glaze:
1. In a saucepan over medium-high heat, reduce figs and balsamic vinegar by three-quarters.
2. Add honey and continue to reduce slowly for 3 minutes. Strain figs and allow glaze to cool.

Pilaf:
1. Heat grapeseed oil in a medium saucepan and add celery, carrot, and shallots.
2. Sweat vegetables for 1 minute, then add quinoa, chicken broth, and bay leaf.
3. Turn heat down and cover pot with foil. Continue to cook for 15 minutes. Remove cooked quinoa from heat and let stand, covered, for 5 minutes. Season with salt and pepper.

Hazelnuts:
1. Preheat oven to 350°.
2. Place hazelnuts on a sheet pan and lightly toast in oven for 4–5 minutes, then set aside.
3. In a sauté pan, add grapeseed oil, rosemary, garlic, and red pepper flakes. Cook over medium heat until oil begins to simmer and garlic and rosemary are lightly toasted.
4. Remove from heat and add toasted hazelnuts and lemon juice. Stir well.

Vanilla Pear Purée:
1. Place pears in a casserole dish. Add shallots, vanilla bean, honey, lemon juice, and butter.
2. Cover with foil and bake in 350° oven for 30 minutes, until tender. Remove vanilla bean and scrape seeds into a blender along with remainder of roasted ingredients. Purée until smooth.

Duck:
1. In a large sauté pan over medium-low heat, lightly season duck breasts with salt and pepper and sear skin-side down 5–7 minutes, until skin is golden brown and crispy.
2. Flip duck over and place in 350° oven for 8–10 minutes. This will yield medium doneness. Remove from oven and let rest. Glaze with Fig-Balsamic Glaze.

To Finish:
1. Warm up quinoa pilaf and place a large spoonful on the plate. Spoon a dollop of purée next to quinoa.
2. Slice duck and arrange on top of quinoa. Sprinkle toasted hazelnuts around the duck and serve.

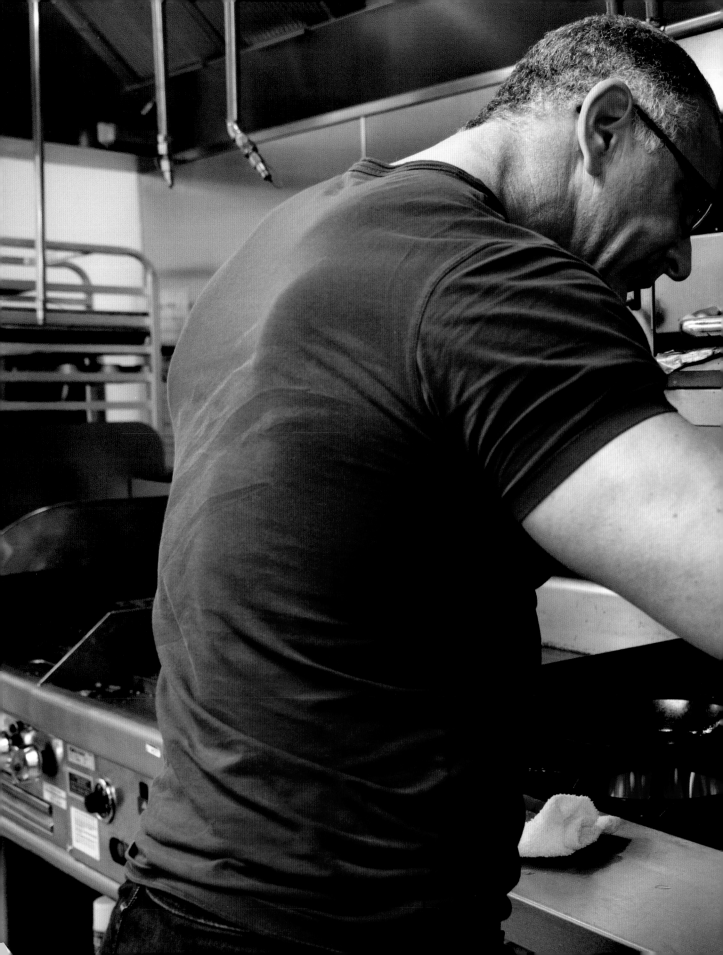

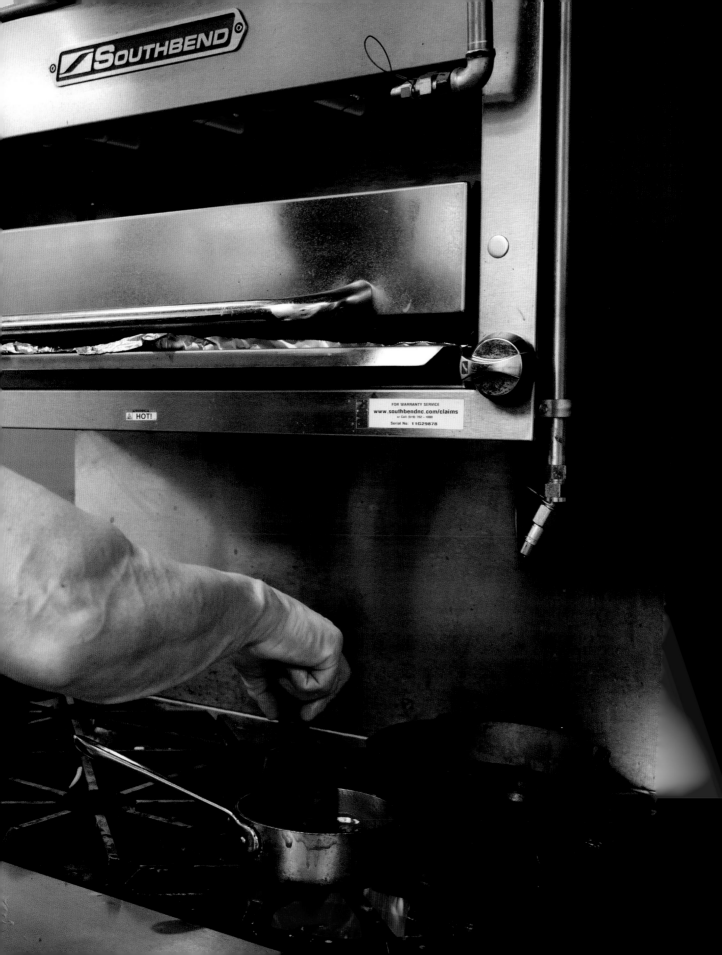

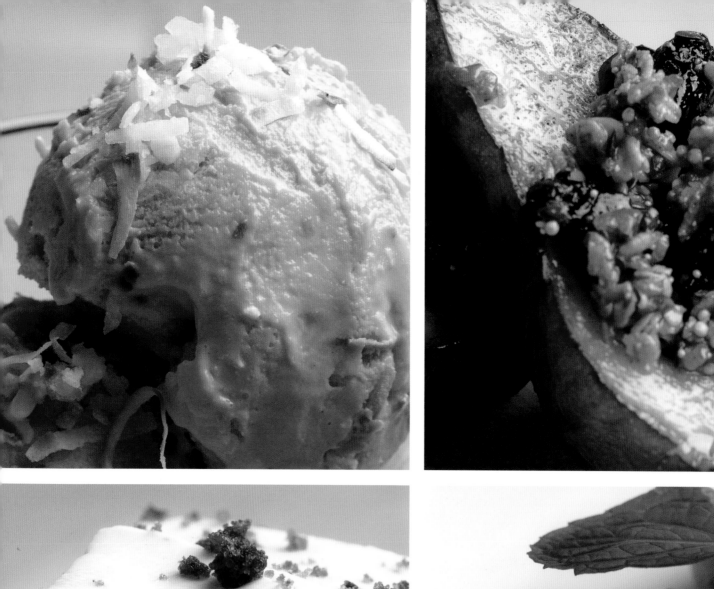
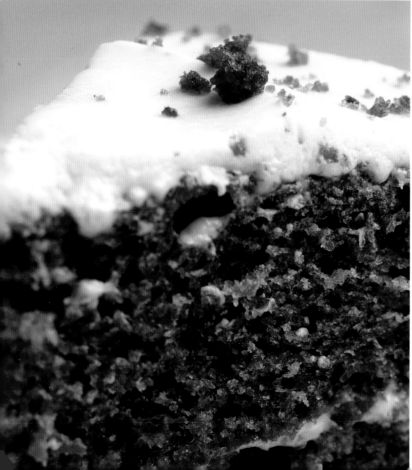
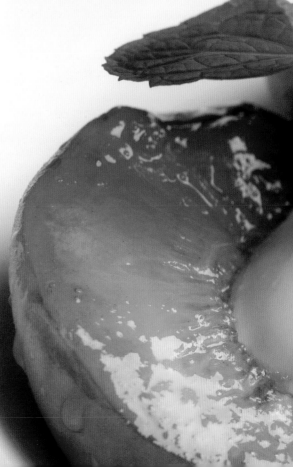

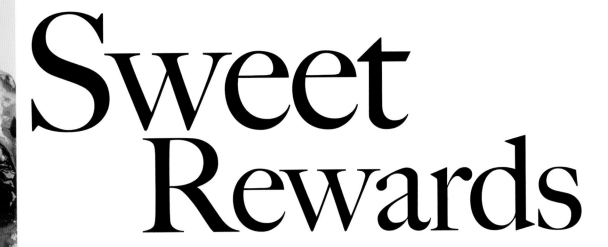

Sweet Rewards

CHEAT MEALS ARE IMPORTANT, not only to save our sanity when we're dieting, but also to refuel our muscles and stoke our metabolism to induce additional fat loss.

However, if you have a lot of weight to lose, you need to be careful with cheat meals. If you go overboard, you can easily undo a ton of hard work. At the same time, a diet without any cheat meals is destined for failure. For most people, one cheat meal per week is a good rule to go by. You can put away the calculator, enjoy a heavy dinner and a decadent dessert one night a week, then get back on track the next day.

For days you're not cheating, consider fruit-based desserts, of which I'm a huge fan. They offer a chance to satisfy your sweet tooth without indulging in a calorically dense pastry. For the carrot cake recipe, save that for a day when you train your absolute hardest, and try to have it within a couple hours after you train. When your muscles are depleted, your body has the ability to use simple sugars and extra calories to restore and repair working muscles. But when you eat heavy, decadent food on an off-day, you're much more likely to store those extra calories as fat.

In any case, these desserts beat the hell out of eating prepackaged, highly processed cookies and candy bars. Making them from scratch, with real, fresh ingredients, is always a better long-term strategy than eating something that came from a factory. Just be sure to enjoy responsibly.

The Menu

Roasted Peaches
with Vanilla Greek Yogurt

Forget peaches and cream. This is a dessert you'll always have room for.

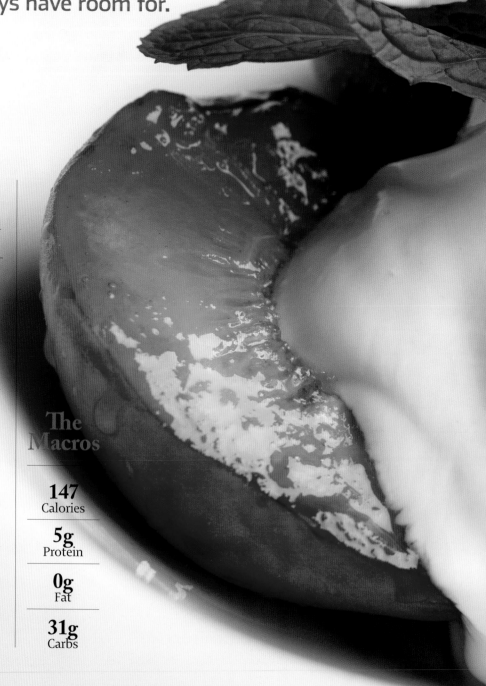

Ideal for: Any Day
Makes 6 Servings

+ YOU'LL NEED

6 tbsp brown sugar

2 dashes salt

4 tbsp Grand Marnier

½ tsp vanilla extract

6 peaches, halved and pitted

2 cups nonfat plain Greek yogurt

1 vanilla bean, split

+ TO MAKE IT

1 Preheat oven to 350°.

2 In a mixing bowl, combine 4 tbsp of the brown sugar, 1 dash salt, Grand Marnier, and vanilla extract. Whisk ingredients together and toss in peaches. Combine until peaches are coated.

3 Place peaches, cut-side up, on a sheet pan lined with parchment paper. Spoon remainder of liquid from bowl onto peaches. Bake for 15 minutes, or until tender. Set peaches aside.

4 Combine yogurt, 2 tbsp brown sugar, vanilla bean seed, and 1 dash salt in a mixing bowl. Mix well.

5 To serve, arrange peaches on a platter and top with Greek yogurt.

The Macros

147
Calories

5g
Protein

0g
Fat

31g
Carbs

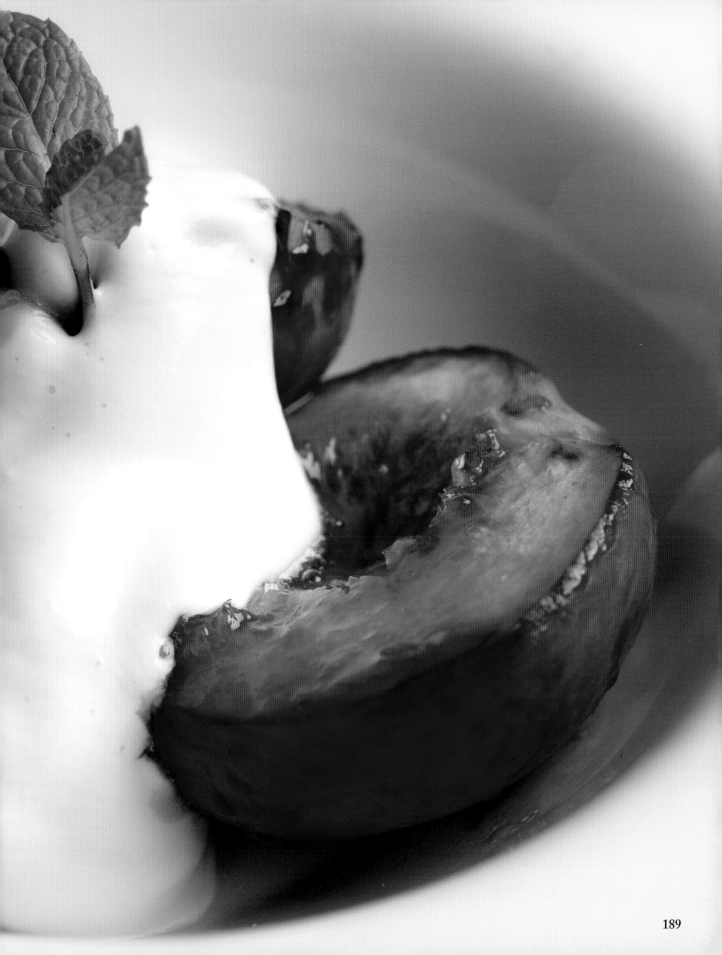

Roasted Pears
with Granola
& Cranberries

Caramelized natural sugars—and a satisfying crunch—put this one over the top.

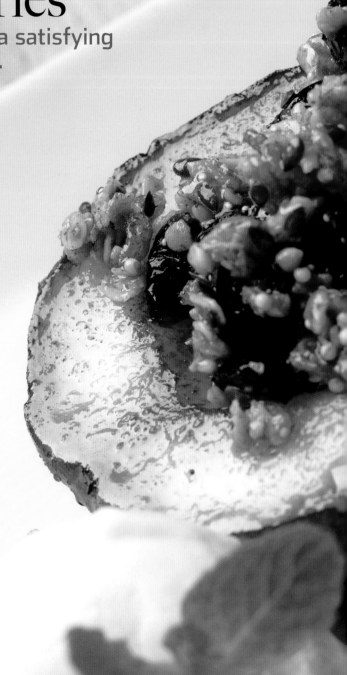

Ideal for: Any Day
Makes 6 Servings

+ YOU'LL NEED

3 pears

3 tbsp stevia

¼ tsp ground cinnamon

½ cup dried cranberries

½ cup low-fat granola

⅓ cup apple juice

1½ cups low-fat vanilla frozen yogurt, divided into 6 scoops

+ TO MAKE IT

1 Preheat oven to 350°.

2 Peel pears and cut in half lengthwise. Scoop out core with a spoon. Place in a glass casserole dish, cut-side up.

3 Combine stevia and cinnamon. Sprinkle on top of pears.

4 Combine dried cranberries and granola in a mixing bowl. Set aside.

5 Pour apple juice into pan with pears.

6 Place pan in oven and bake for 10 minutes. Remove pan and mound the granola/cranberry mixture into the holes created by the missing cores. Return pan to oven and bake for an additional 10 minutes.

7 Remove pan and allow to sit for 5 minutes. Plate pears and drizzle with remaining juice. Serve with frozen yogurt.

The Macros

140
Calories

3g
Protein

1g
Fat

31g
Carbs

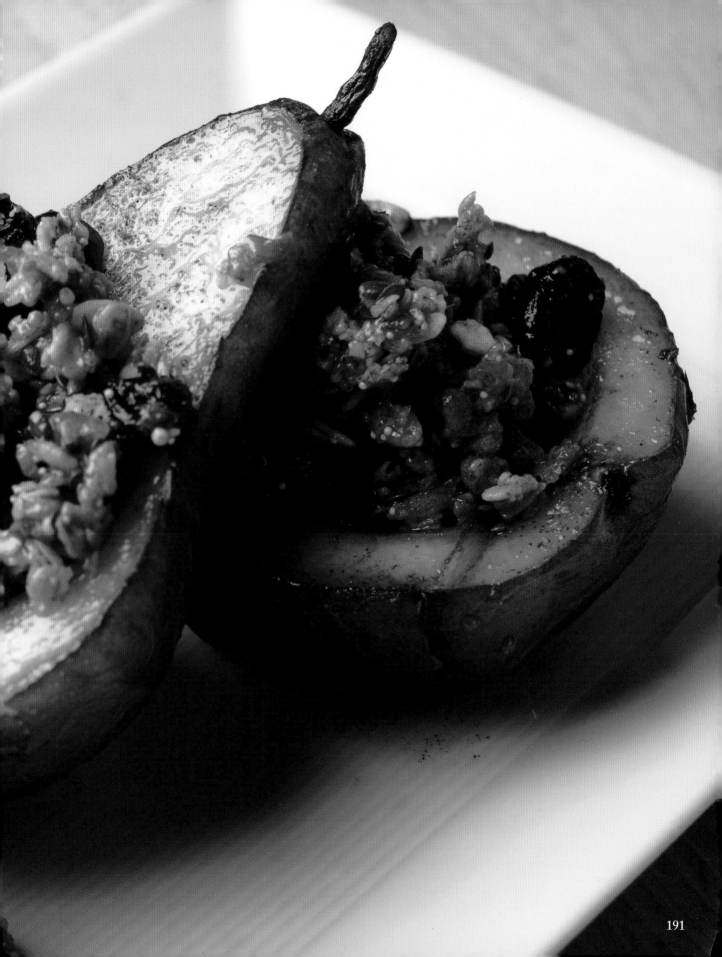

Mango & Toasted Coconut Sorbet

Nothing in the frozen dessert aisle can touch this.

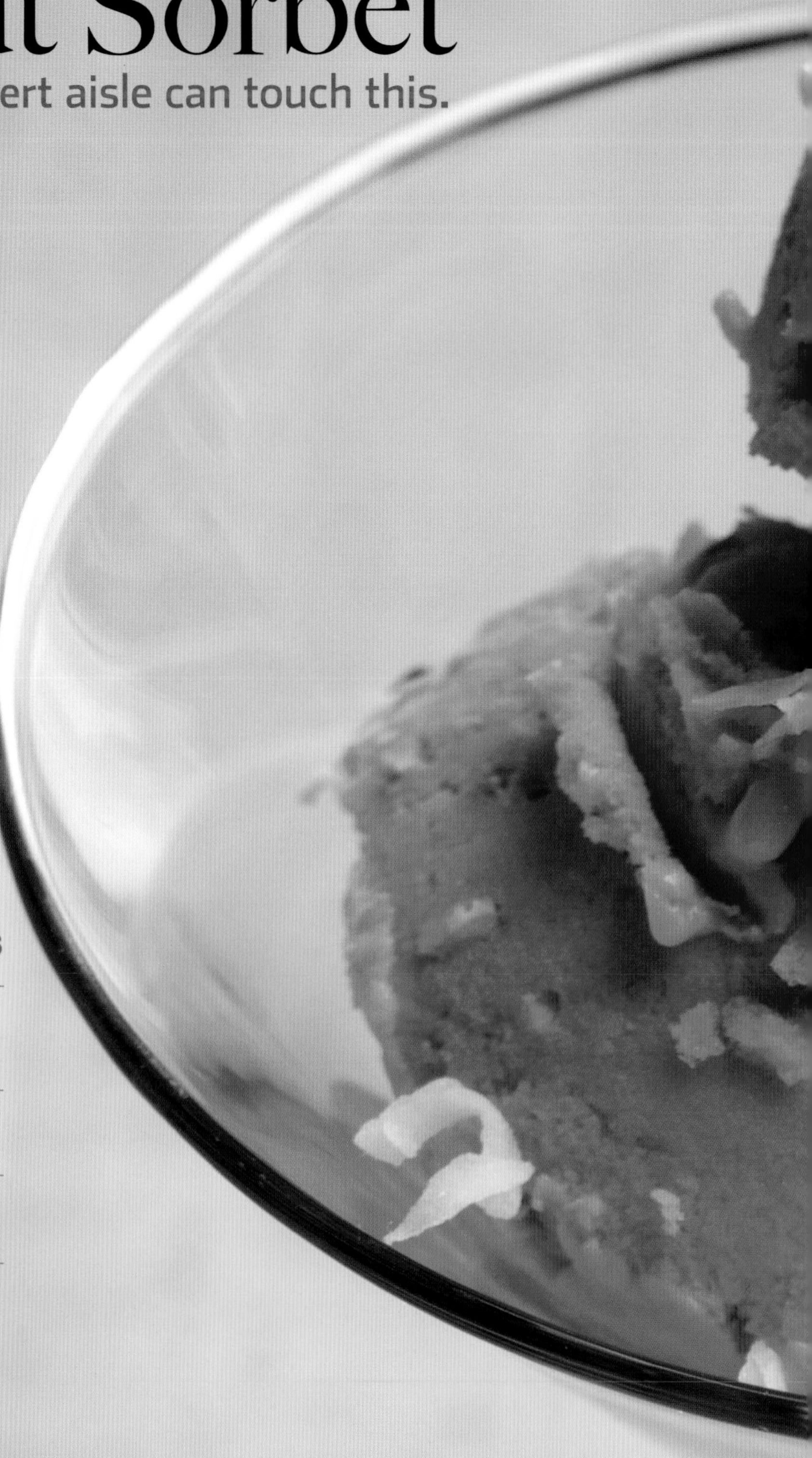

Ideal for:
A Hard
Training Day
Makes 6 Servings

+ YOU'LL NEED

Ice cream maker required
5 ripe mangoes, peeled and pitted

1 cup toasted coconut flakes

Juice of **2** limes

1½ cups water

7 tbsp raw agave nectar

+ TO MAKE IT

1 Combine ingredients in a blender and blend until smooth.

2 Put into ice cream maker for 25 minutes (or time suggested in your ice cream maker's instruction manual).

3 Freeze for at least 3 hours before serving. Top with additional coconut.

The Macros

238
Calories

1g
Protein

5g
Fat

50g
Carbs

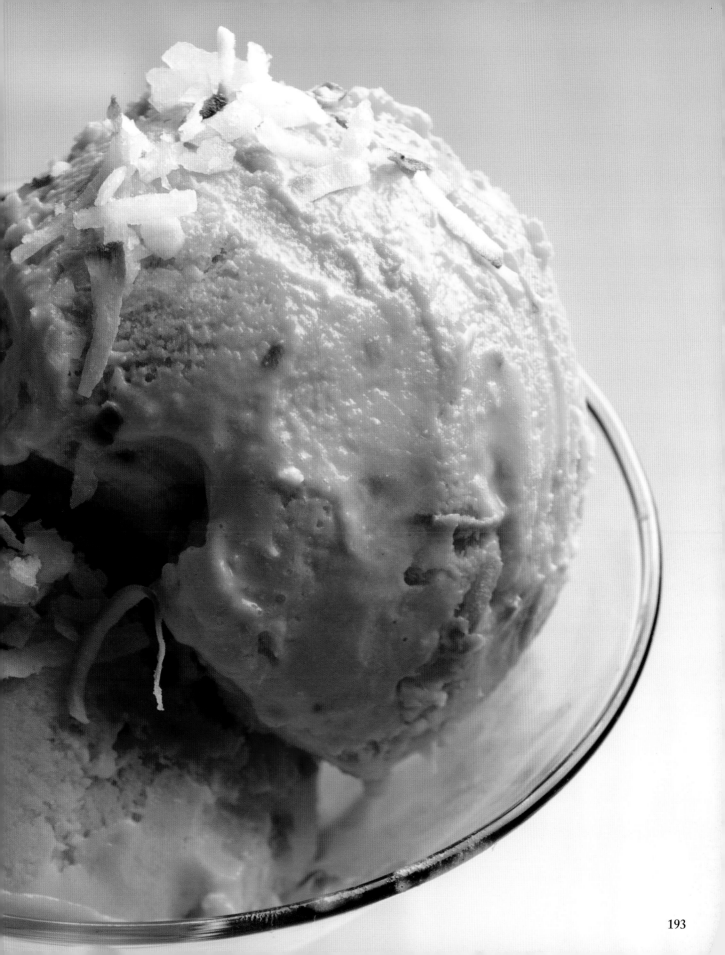

A Better Carrot Cake
The way it was meant to taste.

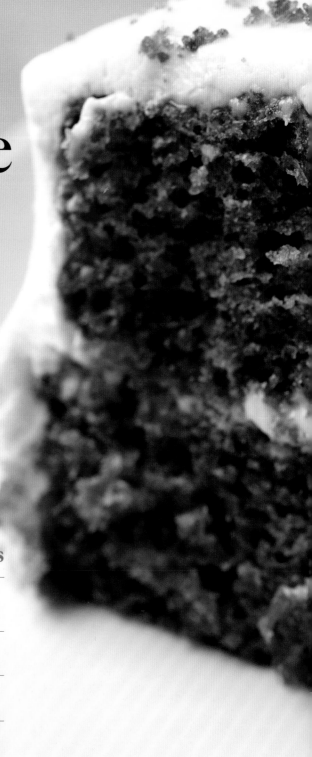

Ideal for: A Cheat Day
Makes 6 Servings

+ YOU'LL NEED

For the Cake:

2 cups whole-wheat flour

¼ cup stevia

2 tsp baking soda

1 1/2 tsp ground cinnamon

½ tsp ground nutmeg

½ tsp salt

¾ cup apple sauce

¼ cup grapeseed oil

3 whole organic eggs

¼ cup skim milk

1 tbsp vanilla extract

3 cups raw carrots, shredded

Nonstick, nonfat cooking spray

For the Frosting:

8 oz low-fat cream cheese

½ cup stevia

1 tsp vanilla extract

+ TO MAKE IT

1 Preheat oven to 350°.

2 In a large mixing bowl, combine all dry ingredients except carrots.

3 In a separate mixing bowl, combine all wet ingredients.

4 Combine wet and dry ingredients and mix well. Add carrots and mix again.

5 Pour batter into a sprayed cake pan and bake for 1 hour.

6 Check cake for doneness by inserting a toothpick into center. If it comes out clean, the cake is done; if it's covered in batter, cook for an additional 7–10 minutes and check again.

7 Remove from oven and allow to rest for 5–10 minutes. Run a butter knife around edges of pan to loosen cake. Place a plate on top of cake pan and turn pan over. Allow cake to continue to cool.

8 Make frosting by beating all frosting ingredients together until soft and smooth. Spread evenly on cooled cake.

The Macros

341 Calories

13g Protein

12g Fat

42g Carbs

The Big Reveal

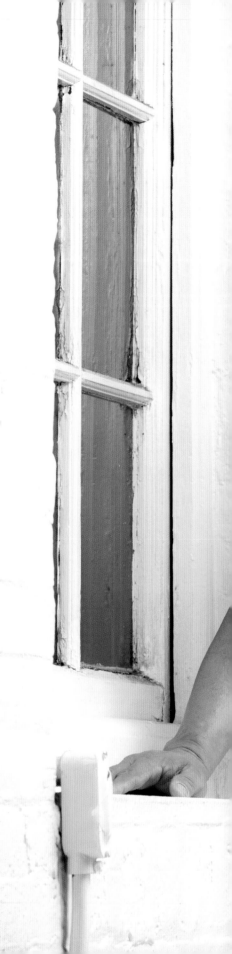

AT THE END OF EVERY EPISODE of *Restaurant: Impossible,* we showed the big reveal. The failing owners closed their eyes and were guided into their newly renovated restaurant. When they opened their eyes, they saw the new décor, the dining room set for new customers lined up outside, and fresh food from their brand-new menu ready to be served. It was always an emotional scene—lots of drama, lots of hugging, lots of crying.

The big difference between you and a failing restaurateur is that no one can come in and renovate for you. No part of your transformation will happen in two short days, either. I've provided the framework for you to get fit—a new training program and menu, with as much encouragement as I could give. What happens from here on out is in your hands.

I hope you've made the commitment to change and are sticking with it. I hope you're training hard and eating right. I hope you've stopped thinking of all the reasons why you can't do it, and replaced those thoughts with visions of getting everything you want out of life: more energy, better health and fitness, and more confidence. However far along you are, I want you to acknowledge how much work you've put into this change so far, applaud yourself for it, and continue to stay the course.

Your own big reveal will come in stages. You'll wake up one morning and you won't feel so tired. Your clothes will start to feel more comfortable and when you get to work, people will compliment you on your appearance. Eventually, you'll step on the scale and see a number that maybe you haven't seen since college or even high school. When people ask you to go to the beach or to a pool, you won't hesitate because you'll be eager to show off what a big change you've made.

Be thankful that you're on a journey where no one can step in and take over a lion's share of the work on your behalf. The beauty of fitness is that in the process of getting physically stronger, we become mentally stronger. Once you've developed the discipline to master your own body and the daily habits that create success, you've not only given yourself a new lease on life, but opened the door to a whole new world of possibilities. Ultimately, fitness is a microcosm of life: If you visualize a goal and commit to it with hard work, faith, and patience, it's yours.

So as you dream, be sure to dream big.

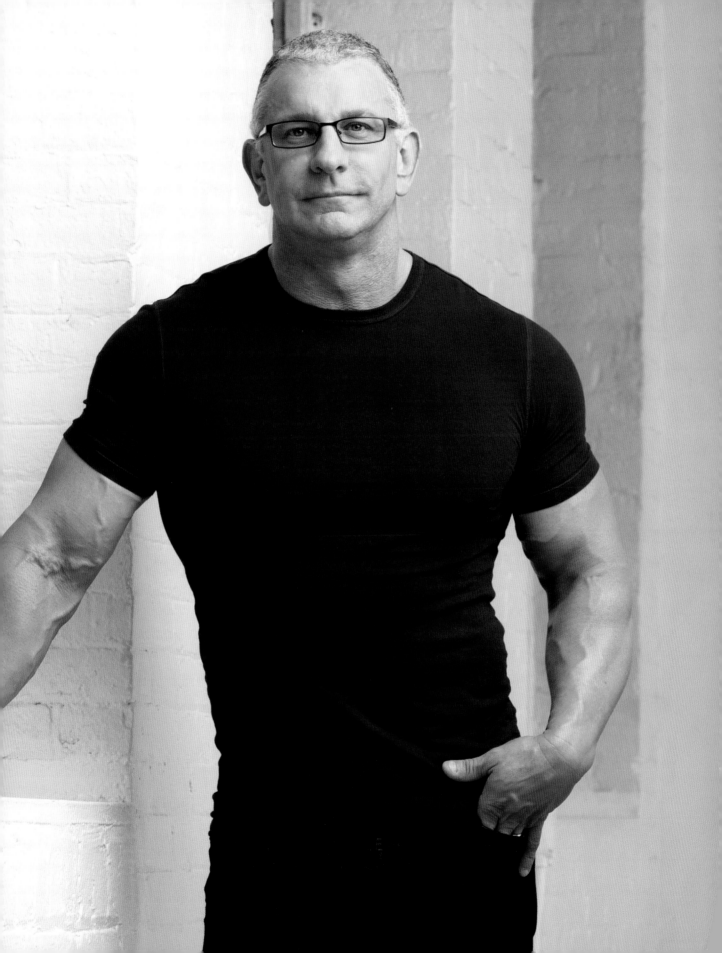

Acknowledgements

Writing this book was a labor of love, and it feels amazing to be able to finally share it with you. The first thank you I'd like to offer is to you, for taking this journey with me.

MAKING *FIT FUEL* A REALITY was not, however, a road I walked alone. A special thank you is owed to my beautiful wife, Gail, who supported this project the way she has every aspect of my career: with love, grace, and patience. You are truly one of a kind. Thank you, Love!

To my daughters, Annalise and Talia, you helped with this book, too, even if you didn't know it! I want to be around for a long time for you—you were huge motivators for me to get healthy and ultimately write a book like this. Thank you! I'm very proud of you both.

A very big thanks goes to my co-author Matt Tuthill, for helping me put my thoughts on paper and working to assemble the team of great talents whose creative energy really made this book pop. Thanks especially to my brilliant Creative Director, Sean Otto, and my peerless photographer, Ian Spanier. *Fit Fuel* looks as good as it does because of you two, and I am in your debt.

Thank you to my Executive Chef, Shane Cash, for helping me develop the recipes in this book and for challenging me creatively every day. To my personal trainer, Hany Rambod, thank you for educating me and pushing me past what I thought was possible at this point in my life.

Thank you to my editors, Nina Combs and Lynette Combs, for their keen eyes for style and flow—and their ability to keep those eyes steady during the long nights finishing *Fit Fuel*. Thank you to my Research Editor, Adam Bible, for double- and triple-checking the science behind every claim made in this book. You're a machine.

Thank you to Dan McLean for your hard work in keeping this project organized and to Justin Leonard and the rest of my team for believing in and supporting everything that I do.

Thank you to Francesca Otto and Jill Tuthill for your valuable input, not to mention for putting your husbands on loan for the completion of this book. Thank you to John Dominioni, Mike Geremia, Daniel Ketchell, John Quinlan, Arnold Schwarzenegger, Chelsea Tuthill, Sherona Varulkar Kelley, and Joseph White for your own unique contributions.

I also owe thanks for the support of Joe DeFranco, Marty Dobrow, John Flanagan, Sean Hyson, David Jeffries, David Scott, Jim Smith, Chris Tuthill, and Libby and Howie Tuthill.

Last but not least, thank you to American Media CEO David Pecker and *Muscle & Fitness* Editor-in-Chief Shawn Perine for giving me a platform to share the concepts behind *Fit Fuel* with the world every month.

You are all world class!

Robert Irvine

Robert Irvine is a celebrity chef best known for his Food Network programs *Restaurant: Impossible* and *Dinner: Impossible.* In addition to his many TV projects, he tours the country for *Robert Irvine Live!* an eclectic, unscripted event that showcases his unparalleled ability to improvise. A veteran of the British Royal Navy, Robert has his own 501c3, the Robert Irvine Foundation, which supports the men and women who defend our country, as well as their families. You can read more about his various projects—which are too numerous to list here—at *chefirvine.com.* Follow him on Twitter: @robertirvine. He lives in Tampa, FL, with his wife, Gail.

Matt Tuthill

Fit Fuel co-author Matt Tuthill is a Certified Physical Preparation Specialist (CPPS) and the Deputy Editor of *Muscle & Fitness* magazine, where he has edited Robert's monthly column since 2011. A former personal trainer, Matt writes features and profiles athletes and celebrities for the magazine. A selected collection of his work can be found at *matt-tuthill.com.* Follow him on Twitter: @MCTuthill. He lives in Rocky Point, NY, with his wife, Jill.

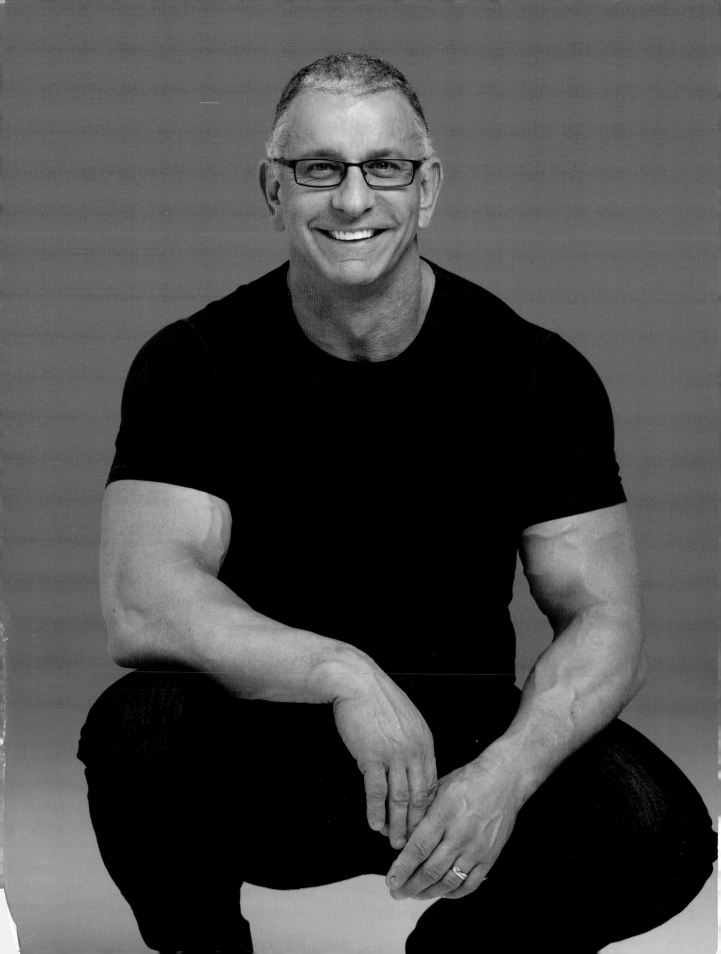